RECOVERY WITH YOGA

RECOVERY
WITH
YOGA

Supportive Practices for
Transcending Addiction

Brian Hyman

Foreword by Tommy Rosen

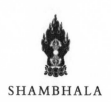

SHAMBHALA

Shambhala Publications, Inc.
2129 13th Street
Boulder, Colorado 80302
www.shambhala.com

Cover art: BD ARMANS/Shutterstock
Cover design: Daniel Urban-Brown
Interior design: Greta D. Sibley

9 8 7 6 5 4 3 2 1

First Edition
Printed in the United States of America

Shambhala Publications makes every effort
to print on acid-free, recycled paper.
Shambhala Publications is distributed worldwide by
Penguin Random House, Inc., and its subsidiaries.

Library of Congress Cataloging-in-Publication Data
Names: Hyman, Brian, author.
Title: Recovery with yoga: supportive practices for transcending addiction
/ Brian Hyman.
Description: First edition. | Boulder, Colorado: Shambhala, [2024]
Identifiers: LCCN 2023011963 | ISBN 9781611809909 (trade paperback)
Subjects: LCSH: Yoga. | Mindfulness-based cognitive therapy. |
Substance abuse—Treatment. | Addicts—Rehabilitation.
Classification: LCC B132.Y6 H88 2024 | DDC 158.1/3—dc23/eng/20230512
LC record available at https://lccn.loc.gov/2023011963

CONTENTS

FOREWORD

If the goal of writing anything is to offer readers the opportunity to experience some kind of revelation, some uplevelling of awareness, and ultimately to be transported and transformed, then Hyman has achieved that here. This work is important and will serve people who are looking to live their best lives in recovery. It is therefore with a sense of gratitude and honor that I write this foreword. I hope to illuminate just exactly how and why this book is so important, and to prepare readers for the gifts that are forthcoming in these pages.

For over three decades, I have been helping people recover from addiction and thrive in life. Yoga and the twelve steps have been the central components of that work. While it was the twelve-step program that laid the foundation for my own recovery, it was the practice of yoga that allowed me to build an extraordinary life on that foundation. Simply put, yoga has given depth and meaning to my recovery and life. I feel it will be helpful and relevant to tell you a bit about my first experiences with yoga to illuminate the most obvious benefit of the physical practice—it feels good. My initial discovery of yoga took place in the summer of 1991, at the very beginning of my recovery. I was walking down the street in San Francisco and saw a large neon sign which read simply, "Yoga." I stepped right into a beginner yoga class that absolutely humbled me. I listened to the teacher, gave it all I had, sweated profusely, and then lay down in savasana (rest pose) at the end of class.

In my book, *Recovery 2.0*, I wrote about this experience: "The feeling was electric—energy humming through my body. I felt like blood was pouring into areas of my tissues that it had not been able to reach for some time. It was relieving and healing. It was subtler than the feeling from getting off on drugs, but it was detectable and lovely, and there would be no hangover, just a feeling of more ease than I could remember. I felt a warmth come over me similar to what I felt when I had done heroin, but far from the darkness of that insanity, this was pure light—a way through."

About a year later, I woke up one morning with an incredible realization: I could not remember the last time I had a thought, much less a craving, about using drugs. What is even more astounding is the fact that in the thirty-one years since then, no thought or craving to use drugs has returned.

I feel that the practice and study of yoga made this possible for me.

Once a person in recovery is turned onto the path of yoga, they gain access to practices and principles that can lead to full recovery and freedom. Yoga provides access to ease in the body, mental calmness, personal empowerment, and self-love. With yoga, a deeper detoxification and a more profound connection to the joy of existence become possible.

The journey of recovery from addiction is a yogic path. Yoga is recovery. Recovery is yoga.

To fully recover from addiction, it takes a holistic and comprehensive approach. One needs certain "vitamins" that are not all found in the work of the twelve steps, nor in psychological processes alone, nor in medical/psychiatric/pharmacological solutions. Yoga is the great medicine, a path of discovery for our modern age that provides the ingredients for healing addiction, which is part of the human condition.

Thus, to read a book that brings together the time-tested practice and philosophy of yoga with the powerful psycho-social-spiritual gifts of modern-day recovery is an incredible pleasure for me. This book will be helpful and perhaps necessary to anyone interested in living their best life in recovery.

Hyman has written a guidebook for the process of yoga-based recovery, which, as noted, is a comprehensive and effective approach to healing addiction.

In *Recovery with Yoga*, Hyman explores thirty powerful concepts, one chapter at a time, fleshing out each one to help readers build a more complete understanding of themselves through the lens of each concept. He threads Yogic teachings into each section, illuminating their deeper meanings, and then he provides questions for reflection at the end of each chapter. *Recovery with Yoga* includes psychology, philosophy, ethics, and practice. It hits the three main dimensions of our being—mind, body, and spirit—and it will also help a person to heal their relationship with time by directing them to that "place where recovery exists"—the present moment.

Thankfully, Hyman is not guiding us toward mere abstinence. He wishes that we experience the fullest possible bloom of our recovery, which is to say, freedom and fulfillment in this life.

This book is an important accompaniment to anyone's recovery journey. If you dive into these pages with earnestness, amazing things will come to pass.

With love and gratitude for all,
Tommy Rosen, author and founder of Recovery 2.0

Introduction

Do you know why you are here? What inspired you to pick up this book? What do you hope to achieve by reading these chapters? Are you interested in learning more about the causes and conditions of addiction? Enhancing your existing program of action for recovery? Learning the value of universal principles? Developing your awareness of spirituality? Discovering how yogic teachings can complement your way of living life?

Unless you have an idea of what you would like to accomplish as the result of the work you will do throughout this book, you will unlikely receive the full benefits such an endeavor can provide. Simply put, you must know your starting point at any given moment in recovery since it does not matter so much where you have been or what you have done in the past but where you are in *the reality of now* and what you plan to do in the present moment if you are to live a meaningful life today and in the future.

The job of any teacher, mentor, sponsor, or therapist who works in recovery is to point you home to your innermost self. All the answers you need are within you. Peace is there. Calm is there. Joy is there. Wisdom is there. Love is there. Recovery is there. This has always been and will always be true. The purpose of this book is to help you return to your authentic, recovered self so you can become the person you are destined to be. The principles and practices in this book will guide and support you as you discover your personal truth, learn to appreciate the precious miracle of life, and fulfill your individual purpose within this lifetime.

Most people in recovery know what it feels like to be disconnected from our deepest truth. We know what it means to lose touch with the inherent health at the center of our being. We are aware of how addiction can devastate our mind, destroy our body, and sever connections to our spirit. Many people who suffer from active addictions and similar issues can remain in pain for years and never find the help we need. We might even refuse to do what ought to be done to become well. And we may ultimately abandon hope and resign ourselves to a life of unending misery and eternal darkness.

However, you are here now and holding this book in your hands. That means you are interested in embarking on a unique inner journey to reclaim your rightful sense of self, reestablish the nature of your sobriety, and revitalize your design for living in recovery. You are determined to do something positive for yourself today. You are willing to do the next right thing to remain healthy and happy. You are ready to deepen your understanding of recovery in order to live the life you are here to live one day at a time.

If you remain open-minded and optimistic, you will find what it is you seek within these pages. If you are diligent and determined as you work through this book, you will come to know your true self. And if you allow your whole heart to guide you throughout this process, you will not only learn about concepts and exercises that enhance recovery and all areas of life but also become empowered to share your experiences with others so you can be a beacon of light to those who have yet to find their true path to wellness.

HOW THIS BOOK CAME TO BE

When I had experienced two months of continuous sobriety, I began to practice yoga every day as part of my personal program of action for recovery. Each time I stepped onto my mat, I learned to breathe consciously and move mindfully, and my mind became quiet and still; my body was purified and strengthened; and I established spiritual contact with a loving and compassionate higher power of my own understanding.

When I was nine months sober, I decided to try to bring the healing and transformative benefits of yoga to others in recovery who didn't know about it or couldn't get to it. I soon completed a yoga teacher training program in Venice, California. Shortly thereafter, I began to teach a free yoga class for people in recovery within the Los Angeles area, which I would continue to do every week for the following two years. I next began teaching yoga classes each week for more than ten years at Cliffside Malibu, a prominent treatment center for addiction recovery in Southern California. I then compiled a list of spiritual principles and yogic practices that had proved beneficial to people in recovery, and based on these teachings, I created the interactive audio course "Recovery: Principles for a Purposeful Life" for the top-rated meditation app Insight Timer.

This book is the culmination of my personal and professional work over the last twelve years. Every chapter summarizes established principles and practices that have healed and transformed my life and the lives of countless others in recovery around the world. And every page provides opportunities to recognize how people in recovery can come home to themselves to find lasting happiness, peace, and freedom.

HOW TO USE THIS BOOK

Set aside what you may know or believe about recovery, yoga, spirituality, and life in general. Be willing to explore the many aspects of these topics so you can develop a new appreciation for all dimensions of the mind, body, and spirit.

Find a quiet place to read this book so that you can have a personal and intimate experience with the material and you can process and internalize your thoughts and reflections as they happen in the present moment without unnecessary disturbances.

Honor your journey as you read through each section of every chapter. Find an individual pace and means by which you can understand all of the material.

Wherever you are in your recovery—remember you are not alone. Many others around the world are also living life in recovery right now and becoming the best and highest version of themselves right now.

Wherever you are today mentally, emotionally, physically, or spiritually—try to find acceptance, contentment, compassion, and love for yourself. Know that you are walking a courageous path.

Be humble as you discover who or what you truly are and freely share what you find with those in need.

1

Honesty

Honesty is the most crucial principle for anyone in early sobriety or recovery. When someone who has a problem with alcohol, drugs, other substances, or similar issues and behaviors can be truly honest with themselves, recovery is inevitable. When someone who suffers from alcoholism, addiction, or related diseases of any kind can admit, claim, or simply tell the truth about what is really going on, this sets the foundation for everything to come.

There is a quote about honesty that has been attributed to the Buddha: "Three things can't remain hidden long—the sun, the moon, and the truth." It would seem that whether we like it or not, just as the sun and moon will rise and be seen, the truth will also rise and be seen.

How do we process what needs to be processed before the truth rises? How do we name and own our truth? What is the inner work we need to do to figure out our truth? How are we to heal our truth before it is revealed? Is there something we are trying to hide? And if so, why?

Before we answer these questions, let's look at why we might be afraid to answer them. There is often shame attached to things we do when we are stuck in the regularity of active addiction. There is often painful trauma buried in the consciousness of people who use and abuse substances. There is often immeasurable embarrassment in the hearts of those who experience prolonged states of disease. There is often deep remorse, guilt, and regret in the mind of the alcoholic, addict, and others who suffer from these types of conditions.

Honesty in recovery requires us to acknowledge the things we would rather forget. It would call us to take one contrary action after another: forgo what our ego or pride would have us believe; expose our weaknesses to others without attachment to the results. We would need to open our mind and heart to humility and humanity. We would need to bring negative, dark, and uncomfortable things out in the open. We would need to confess inner and outer wrongs. We would need to trust that honesty can deliver us from disease to wellness and from the uncertainty of addiction to the reliability of recovery.

A MOMENT OF TRUTH

In November 2009, I began to attend twelve-step meetings each morning in Los Angeles. I had not yet identified as an alcoholic, nor told anybody why I was at the meetings. I sat alone in the back rows of these rooms. I kept my head down. I did not speak to anyone.

One morning near the beginning of a meeting, a speaker asked if any newcomers or anyone in their first thirty days of sobriety wished to identify themselves. If so, they were encouraged to raise a hand, say their name, and mention why they were there.

There was a long pause. Then one person near the back of the room raised his hand. He said his name and that he was an alcoholic. The group repeated his name, clapped their hands, and welcomed him. Then another person near the front of the room raised her hand. She said her name and that she was an alcoholic and a drug addict. The group repeated her name, clapped their hands, and welcomed her. Then the room was quiet.

Something in my chest began to tremble. My legs began to shake. My heart started to race. I felt hot and sweaty. My vision seemed cloudy. Something wretched seemed to move up through my insides to get outside. Without a conscious thought, my hand shot into the air. I said my name and that I was an alcoholic. The group repeated my name, clapped their hands, and welcomed me.

I stopped shaking and sweating. My heart rate returned to normal. Tears filled my eyes. The secret that I kept hidden for decades had finally been set free. An older gentleman next to me placed his hand on my shoulder. He whispered: "Welcome."

I could not remember another time in my life when I felt that accepted. Or broken. Or broken open. Or honest.

I have had many years to reflect on that morning. I have wondered why I was finally honest about something I believed made me inferior, broken, and worthless; why the time for honesty had come despite my fears about what might happen next; why the truth about a sickness that had been locked inside me for years was irreversibly released.

I have yet to find answers to these questions. I have instead accepted the idea that it was time for me to leave behind the energy of addiction forever and rise up to another level of being. It was time for me to know a freedom I had never known. It was time for me to do something meaningful with the precious gift of life.

THE TRUTH ABOUT ADDICTION

Addiction is no respecter of persons, titles, riches, pedigree, or power. It does not care if it destroys families or communities. It does not care if it maims or kills. It seeks one thing: complete devotion.

Addiction wants us to bow down to it. It wants our undivided attention. It will do anything to keep us in denial. It will do anything to make sure we are forever its prey.

Addiction uses dishonesty as a weapon to alter our thoughts, words, and actions. It employs deceit, confusion, fiction, and other manifestations of untruth to ensure we remain its loyal subjects. It engages treachery, justification, indignation, and equivalent methods to suppress any natural urges we have toward sincerity. It does whatever it can to prevent us from aligning with our inner-most truth.

When we are honest and admit what is seared upon our heart, we become empowered. When we tell the truth, we are no longer confined to the smallness and suffocation of falsehoods.

When we use whatever words we can to share our stories, we are unshackled from the captivity that is addiction and step into a purposeful life in recovery.

Honesty annihilates the bonds of addiction. Honesty informs addiction that we are no longer its slaves. It lets addiction know we will no longer be complicit in manufacturing misery within our lives. Honesty is our ticket to freedom.

When we can't be honest, our mental, emotional, physical, and spiritual health suffers. When we can't tell the truth, we won't know wholeness or wellness. When we remain silent about what is happening within our lives, we will not comprehend the miracles of healing, transformation, or recovery. When we can't be authentic, addiction remains the victor.

DISCOVERING AND PRACTICING HONESTY

Religious, spiritual, and secular traditions present honesty and truth as interchangeable key concepts to be learned and lived if we are to know peace and freedom. In the Bible we are taught: "The truth shall set you free." In the Bhagavad Gita, a sacred Hindu scripture, we are taught: "It is better to die while living your own truth than to live in the truth of another." Even scientists, mathematicians, and engineers confirm the necessity of truth through verifiable facts, formulas, and similar concepts.

Within the Yoga Sutras of Patanjali, an ancient collection of nearly two hundred Sanskrit aphorisms on the theory and practice of yoga for self-realization, *satya* is offered as the moral code of honesty by which we can rightly navigate our lives. The Sanskrit root word *sat* means "truth." Satya is how we are honest in the world. It is how we abide in an authentic place of neutrality. It reveals our communal, timeless, undeniable reality. It constitutes the essence of our inmost being. It is the force by which fluctuations within the mind are calmed, physical reactions become embodied, and spiritual objectives reach maturation.

When we embrace satya as a guiding principle for recovery, our presence is infused with honor, dependability, and righteousness; mistruths no longer originate from within us; our thoughts, words, and deeds benefit the welfare of all beings everywhere; and what we need comes to us as a result of our constitution.

Within the Brihadaranyaka Upanishad, a yogic text that explains the metaphysics of matter and energy, the dynamics of selfhood, and similar universal topics, the Pavamana mantra provides a blueprint to acquiring and harnessing the simplicity and wisdom of satya. Enlightened masters, spiritual aspirants, secular students, and seekers of all types have used the Pavamana mantra for thousands of years to find honesty, transformation, recovery, and much more.

The Sanskrit word *mantra* can be defined as that which protects the mind from things such as errant thoughts, limiting beliefs, regretful reflections, and catastrophized projections—all of which can lead to addiction, depression, anxiety, and other maladaptive behaviors. Let's examine the Pavamana mantra below to understand how it relates to recovery.

> *Om asato ma sadgamaya*
> *Tamaso ma jyotir gamaya*
> *Mrtyor ma amrtam gamaya.*
> *Om shanti, shanti, shanti.*

From untruth lead us to Truth
From darkness lead us to Light
From death lead us to Immortality.
Om, peace, peace, peace.

When we begin with the invocation *Om*, we call out to God, the cosmos, or the divine nature within all things. When we utter the syllable or word *Om*, we find humility. We admit we are unwilling to continue our search for salvation unaccompanied or with personal, limited resources as our only defense. We ask for assistance, kinship, and protection. We renounce our mortal, fallible thoughts. We request and become willing to receive wisdom and strength from a power greater than ourselves.

When we ask to be led from untruth to truth, veils of ignorance will be lifted from our eyes. We will be released from the curse of addiction, and the blessing of recovery will become available to us. We will move from the phenomenal world of unreality toward union with the eternal self. We will be shown how to travel from the awareness of addiction to the insight of recovery.

When we ask to be led from darkness to light, negative patterns of behavior will be replaced by intuitive thoughts and beneficial actions. We will no longer grope through the darkness of active addiction. The glow of spiritual knowledge will illuminate a path toward our inner teacher. Fear will be removed from us and love will guide this process of transfiguration.

When we ask to be led from death to immortality, the gifts of timelessness and freedom will be laid at our feet. We will no longer be addicted to things that bind or imprison us. We will no longer maintain a poverty consciousness or lack mentality. We will see things from a higher perspective. We will be released from personal attachment to transitory things like money, property, and prestige. We will experience the mystical reality of heaven on Earth, the Pure Land of the Buddha, and Mahananda, or ultimate bliss.

When we finish the mantra with the words *Om shanti, shanti, shanti,* we express a wish for individual and collective peace within the thoughts, words, and actions of all beings everywhere. We ask for peace within the trinity of mind, body, and spirit. We attain peace within the realms of past, present, and future.

By whichever means you choose to observe this mantra, set and adhere to an intention to know more about honesty and recovery. Become willing to grasp the meaning of the mantra experientially rather than intellectually. Find your own rhythm and resonance for recitation of this mantra. Internalize your reactions. Use the Sanskrit or English version, or try out another language. Say it once or as many times as desired. Sing it, write it, read it, or locate a recording and listen to it. Remain open-minded to the ideas that will arise.

BEING HONEST WITH OURSELVES

Honesty preserves soundness of mind, body, and spirit. It transforms disease into ease. It creates and patrols an impenetrable perimeter around our recovery. When we rightfully interact with honesty in its myriad forms, the mind and heart are altered and our way of being in the world is revolutionized.

We must practice honesty until it becomes natural, or we will never know the richness of recovery. We must practice honesty if we are to know individual and collective autonomy, harmony, and peace. We must become united with honesty if we are to live our purpose and encourage others to do the same.

Honesty permeates everything. It is unmistakable and invincible. It moves freely throughout time and space. It seeks, finds, and perpetuates itself through thoughts, words, and actions. For example, if we become overwhelmed by emotion when we hear an authentic piece of music, read a riveting passage within a book, or witness a captivating dance performance, it is the honesty within all these things that has touched the honesty within our own hearts.

Active addiction is a constrictive, suffocating, painful prison within which we are unlikely to see, hear, or feel anything but unbearable darkness. It is a living hell built upon the cornerstone of dishonesty.

Recovery is an expansive, receptive, and boundless way of being, by which we accurately perceive reality with all our senses, and our lives become illumined by the light of hope and reason. It is a promise of contentment and inspiration built upon the foundation of honesty.

Honesty begins within the mind as a decision to be a better and kinder person. It begins when we no longer wish to suffer the consequences of dishonesty. It grows one instance at a time, one confession at a time, and one day at a time.

Without honesty there is no escape from addiction. We will not travel far in life. We will not know success, happiness, or joy. We will not become the men and women we are destined to be. Without honesty, the heart will not know true peace; the mind will not know true rest; the body will not know true equanimity. Without honesty, we will unlikely maintain recovery.

LET'S MAKE THIS PERSONAL

Whether you suffer from alcoholism, addiction, or another illness; you have a family member or friend in trouble; or you are just curious about honesty or satya, read the questions below. Pause between them to notice your reactions. Write down your answers and share your responses with a sponsor, therapist, or friend. Allow these questions to highlight areas in your life where you can practice the principle of honesty. Cultivate a personal relationship with honesty.

Do you believe you have a problem with alcohol, drugs, pornography, gambling, food, shopping, work, or something else?

Are you ready to do something positive about troublesome areas in your life?

Are you willing to be honest about something you have never looked at before in a truthful way?

Are you living your purpose?

Is your career fulfilling?

What would you do differently with your life if time and money were not obstacles?

Are you in the right romantic or similar personal relationships?

Are there things you can do differently to be a better employee? Or better spouse? Or better parent? Or better friend?

Is there something in your heart right now that needs to be expressed? If so, what are you waiting for?

What are you willing to admit in order to release a limiting belief?

How can you best embrace your unique purpose or identity within your heart?

What are some ways to better nourish your mind, body, and spirit?

Can you choose a different course of action the next time you become aware of an opportunity to be dishonest?

How can you learn to listen and speak from the heart?

Are there any stories you tell yourself that are no longer true?

2

Acceptance

Acceptance in recovery is becoming aware of any aspect of our lives as truthful. It means recognizing the certainty of something. It is an acknowledgment of whatever is in front of us when it is there.

Acceptance means that we honor the legitimacy of a situation without trying to manipulate the circumstances to appease personal likes or dislikes. It is a neutral evaluation without a positive or negative charge. Allowing what is in front of us to be what it is allows us to take the formal step to recalibrate our awareness so that recovery becomes possible.

We do not need to approve, condone, or appreciate things in order to consider accepting them. We do not need to feel satisfied before we accept something as true. We do not need to feign optimism or make peace with something before we allow accept-ance. When we accept what is, we no longer fight the authenticity of the present moment; we instead move toward solutions that may positively alter our lives and the lives of those around us; we no longer fight old ideas, conditioned behaviors, habit energies or avoid people, places, and things that may benefit recovery.

Acceptance is hardly an easy notion to incorporate into all areas of life, especially when we are attempting to accept the feelings or emotions that arise in addiction or recovery, such as brokenness, worthlessness, hopelessness, self-loathing, or fear. It can be difficult to be open to accepting memories and experiences that bring about shame or regret. It can be difficult to allow that we may have hurt others and ourselves while drunk or during a blackout. It can be difficult to accept anything that paints an unflattering portrait of who or what we become in the grips of ad-diction. However, acceptance leads to sovereignty. It transitions us from one mindset to another. It is how we encounter and transcend commonplace, exceptional, and seemingly impossible situations. It is natural, and in many cases, necessary.

For example, imagine a person is driving a car and the fuel tank is nearly empty. With acceptance, the driver will obtain more fuel and complete the journey. If the driver continues without refilling the tank, the vehicle will likely stall, the driver may become stranded, and the destination will remain out of reach.

Imagine another person is diagnosed with cancer. With ac-ceptance, a proper plan for treatment can be mapped out and implemented. However, if this person remains in denial about the prognosis, they will be unlikely to comply with medical advice, pain will not be alleviated, and healing and remission can't occur.

Now, imagine a person suffers from addiction or similar conditions. With acceptance, this person can get help, work a program of action, and find recovery. If the nature of the problem is rejected or ignored, this person will likely suffer deterioration of the mind, destruction of the body, disconnection from the spirit, and recovery will not be possible.

SEPARATION FROM EGO

If we are to survive addiction and enrich our lives in recovery, we must disassociate from any negative thought patterns and false narratives deterring us from acceptance. We must discover and embrace our true, inner nature to be restored to health. Ultimately, we must rid ourselves of self-interest by diminishing our ego-identification.

Within the yogic tradition, the term *ahamkara* refers to the ego and its ability to create a sense of self-identity through self-serving storytelling. Ahamkara is a state of confusion that disconnects us from the wholesome nature of our identity. Ahamkara leads us to believe that we can edit negativity, shortcomings, and uncomplimentary details from the history of our lives. Ahamkara—a mistaken view of self that separates us from truth—is the major barrier to acceptance.

When ahamkara becomes the lens through which we view addiction, the ego won't allow us to accept anything that does not fit the narrative it wishes to present. When we fall prey to this trick of ego, we become hypnotized by the false idea that ambiguity outperforms truth. When ego orders our affairs, we reject anything that makes us appear weak or wrong; we avoid external aid or support. If we can't override the structure of the ego to accept ourselves and our circumstances, recovery will elude us.

LET'S MAKE THIS PERSONAL

Can you accept that the sky is blue? That the ocean is deep? That trees are green? That flowers bloom?

Can you accept that gravity is proven and functional? Can you accept that rain pours down onto the earth from above? Can you accept that the sun rises and sets?

Can you accept that blood flows throughout the human body? That the heart beats within the chest? That the lungs allow us to breathe?

Can you accept that when dishes get dirty, they ought to be cleaned? When clothes get soiled, they ought to be washed? When a garden is overrun with weeds, it ought to be pruned?

Most likely, you were able to answer yes to most, if not all, of these questions. When we accept things that are correct and reliable, there is no need to feel betrayed, angry, or disappointed. When we accept facts, judgment is hardly necessary, and no arguments or justifications are required.

Now, let's make this a little more personal: Can you accept the nature of your addiction? Can you accept that you may have a problem with a substance or specific behavior? Can you accept that you may need help?

Can you accept that someone you care about may have a problem with addiction? That they may need help? That they are sick or scared?

Can you accept that we are worthy of redemption? That our mess can become our message of hope for others? That our problems can give our lives purpose?

Can you accept that recovery is available to you in the present moment? Can you accept that recovery is available to anyone who desires it?

What were your answers to these questions? Which feelings or emotions emerged from within you as a result of being honest about these topics? When we accept that addiction is part of our lives, we are freed from the burdens of suppression and inauthenticity. When we accept that we have an issue with addiction, we can ascertain the truth about our disease and recognize its attributes and consequences, and in so doing, the mind and heart are transformed.

Remember, the ego fights to protect a falsified image of self. It ignores facts and censors the truth to maintain that image. It brainwashes anyone who threatens its existence. It poisons anything that opposes it. Acceptance short-circuits ego and doesn't allow it to mediate our consciousness to create a false picture of who we are. It allows us to know our inner calm, balance, and peace that come from accepting what is without arguments of justification. And that is the beginning of healing and restoration.

PRACTICING ACCEPTANCE

The following affirmations assist with the process of acceptance. These sentences can be read each morning or evening to boost morale and encourage perception of things as they are. These words honor the human journey from addiction to recovery.

Find your own pace and style of reading these lines. And feel free to adapt this exercise in any way that works best for you.

> I am a human being.
> I am not perfect.
> I make mistakes.
> I do my best.

> I am worthy of love.
> I am on a path to wellness.
> I imagine myself healthy and whole.
> I send thoughts of healing to myself and to
>   anyone who suffers.

> My inner nature is calm, balance, and peace.
> A wellspring of wisdom resides within me.
> Recovery is possible for me today through the
>   power of acceptance.

3

Surrender

When stuck in active addiction, many individuals feel like prisoners. Whether the addiction is alcohol, drugs, sex, gambling, food, shopping, or something else, our personal power hardly proves adequate for our defense or salvation. When we attempt to liberate ourselves from the oppression of addiction and its ancillary habits or consequences, our efforts to establish authority are typically futile.

Consider these questions: If we wish to release ourselves from the bewilderment and pain of addiction, why then do so many alcoholics or addicts continue to drink and use drugs? If we wish to cease injurious behaviors while in the throes of any addiction, why then do we continue to harm ourselves and others? If we wish to achieve continuous recovery, why then is it nearly impossible on our own power?

There is an idea expressed often within addiction recovery circles: If our best thinking gets us into trouble, our best thinking can't get us out of trouble.

Surrender in recovery means that we renounce our finite intelligence, strength, and resources. It means we recognize that our individual efforts are impractical and ineffective, and our personal plans and solutions bring no lasting benefit. It means we are willing to ask for and accept help from a source of power exceeding our own.

A YOGIC PERSPECTIVE OF SURRENDER

Within the Yoga Sutras of Patanjali, the concept of *Isvara pranidhana* is presented as one of five self-disciplines, or *niyamas*. *Isvara* can be translated as "God"; it can also be viewed as supreme consciousness, divine source, or absolute reality. *Pranidhana* is to surrender, devote, or fix our gaze upon. *Isvara pranidhana* is recognized as self-surrender—to God, to humanity, or to a greater good.

When we consider Isvara pranidhana as it relates to recovery, we can empty ourselves of all things, good and bad. We can offer the entirety of our thoughts, memories, and feelings; our words, actions, and character. We can release attachment to the past, present, and future. We can submit ourselves to the process of renewal through complete renunciation of self.

When we practice Isvara pranidhana as part of recovery, we will no longer be restricted by personal frailties or temptations. We will never again face insurmountable inner or outer challenges alone. We will be open to a deep connection to humanity, nature, and the inmost spirit or soul within all things. We will accept the integral role we are destined to play within this lifetime. We will become divinely inspired.

LEARNING TO SURRENDER

When people in active addiction believe that surrendering means giving up or losing something, recovery will be difficult to achieve. When surrender is viewed as a sign of weakness or cowardice, our mental, emotional, and physical energies become depleted in fighting against it. When surrender is deemed impossible because the results may be unpredictable, recovery will not manifest. However, when surrender is viewed as the act of giving oneself up into the power of something superior, troubles fall away and a chosen source of strength commandeers a path to recovery.

Surrender is not nihilistic; it is instead a life-giving choice we take of recognizing the limits of our own power to avoid the precariousness and misery of addiction. It is allowing trust in a power greater than our own to guide us without error through recovery. Surrender can't be forced onto us; we have free will and can choose to destroy or save our lives. Surrender does not mark the end of addiction; it is the beginning of a purposeful life in recovery and beyond.

Surrender is not a new concept for people who have suffered from active addiction. For example, when we are in the grips of addiction, we likely already surrender our ability to be right-minded and honest, to be good parents and responsible friends, to be trustworthy and respectable. We likely surrender our morals and obligations, judgments and feelings, determination and purpose. We likely surrender to fear, selfishness, anger, retribution, apathy, and anxiety. We likely surrender our will to live and thrive. And we likely surrender our capacity to know healing, transformation, and recovery.

Below are suggestions for people in active addiction who may not know how to begin the process of surrender. These ideas are also beneficial for those who feel stuck within their program of recovery.

Reflect on your religious and spiritual beliefs. For example, does your personal idea of God give you a sense of security and strength? If not, do you feel a connection to another deity, avatar, guru, enlightened master, inspirational figure, or concept in your life? Find something that feels right to you and establish conscious contact through devotional or dedicated practices such as prayer and meditation.

Think about universal qualities that are omnipotent, omniscient, and omnipresent. For example, love, truth, intelligence, and similar fundamental principles are ones we can consider eternally reliable. Think of how you can align your thoughts, speech, and actions in accordance with ideals like these.

Within yogic philosophy, the term *atman* describes our highest or innermost self. This is a place of inner knowing at the center of our being where we are perfect and whole. This is where the soul abides; where we are already awakened, healthy, and connected to all sentient things. Cultivate awareness of the atman through silence and complementary introspective practices.

Consider any animate entity that can accomplish something you can't do on your own power—for example, the sun or moon, an ocean, a special tree, a favorite river, a particular mountain. You can also choose an inanimate object that holds special meaning for you, such as a family heirloom or precious keep-sake that reminds you of higher qualities and points you toward mindful thoughts and right actions.

Note: When you choose a personal concept of God or con-template surrender, it is not necessary to explain or justify your decisions. You don't need to convince others of the legitimacy of your beliefs or debate the direction of your recovery. If you feel connected to something higher and attempt to no longer rely on your own power to solve your problems, your ideas of God and surrender will effectively direct you.

SURRENDER AS A WAY OF BEING

Surrender in recovery is a quiet and humble yet mighty act that nourishes emotional well-being, enriches intellectual under-standing, and spiritually unites those on similar paths of dis-covery. It grants us permission to be human and fallible, to remain teachable and maintain the mind of a beginner. It allows us to discard inclinations toward perfectionism so that we are no longer manufacturers of misery but makers of miracles as a higher wisdom directs our affairs.

Surrender must be both a resolute decision and a commit-ment to action for benefits to be received, as surrender is never a means to absolve us of effort. For example, if a person in a twelve-step program surrenders to God or a higher power, they ought to continue to attend meetings, read and study pertinent literature, and remain connected to others in the program.

Surrender is a continual process of rebirth when we hold no reservations about what will happen in our lives as the result of this release and its subsequent actions. Just as waves surrender back into the ocean, we must routinely surrender our will to that which animates our consciousness, often and in earnest.

When surrender becomes a foundational aspect of our lives, we will feel unburdened, hopeful, and composed. We will accurately perceive reality. Our existence will become ordered. We will become approachable and cooperative. We will hardly suffer from paranoia, humiliation, or fatigue. Opportunities to love and serve others will be bestowed upon us. We will be delivered from the battlefield of addiction to the refuge of recovery.

LET'S MAKE THIS PERSONAL

What does surrender truly mean for you today? Is there a specific area of your life where you ought to stop fighting? Where you struggle with what ought to happen next? Where your best efforts fail you?

Where in your life are you willing to try something new or accept help from another source of strength or power? Where are you trying too hard to hold on to things as they are? Where are you failing to create long-lasting change? Where are you losing something you don't want to lose? Would it be possible for you to let go of control and accept help?

Take a few moments and think about these questions. Close your eyes and meditate on thoughts that may arise as a result of your answers. Perhaps write down your reflections in a notebook. Pause to notice the quality of your mind as you contemplate surrender. Notice how your body feels when you think about letting go of control. Notice how your heart or spirit feels when you consider the concept of God or an ultimate source of strength.

4

Courage

When I was a teenager, I portrayed the Cowardly Lion in a school production of the play *The Wizard of Wonderland*. Within this story, the Cowardly Lion desperately desires courage and embarks on an outward journey to find it. After a matinee performance for a group of children, I was asked if the Cowardly Lion truly found his courage and where it really comes from. I was not sure how to answer those questions at the time.

How would you respond to these questions today? Do you think courage can be found by those who seek it? Where do you think it comes from? Do you believe it is something we can find inside ourselves? Or is an outward search necessary?

Let's look at the Sanskrit word *kshatriya*, which means warrior or protector. Kshatriyas can be identified by battle scars on the front of the body, as they never turn from an enemy nor succumb to fear.

Would you consider this true courage? Is it the ability to face fear or opposition without hesitation? Is it to charge forward without attachment to an outcome? Is it to conquer enemies on any path with brute strength? Would this be the best way to overcome addiction?

The courage of a lion or heroism of a warrior can help us achieve sobriety, as bodily force typically affects a target even if desired results are temporary or incomplete. But physical courage and its outward manifestations can't sustain lasting recovery, as transformation requires additional contributions from the emotional, mental, and spiritual realms of our being.

Let's explore these three inwardly potent forms of courage that can fortify our recovery.

EMOTIONAL COURAGE

When we acknowledge and face what lies beneath addiction, such as underlying conditions, family-of-origin issues, or low self-worth, a solid foundation is created for recovery. Hardly anyone enjoys emotional self-examination, but this is essential if we are to achieve freedom from the bondage of chemical dependence or addiction.

If we can't ascertain *why* we do what we do at the level of feeling, we will not be able to stop or alter behaviors that are leading to misery and misfortune. If we can't explore the subtler levels of existence, we will not be able to excavate and harmonize the detrimental causes and conditions leading to addiction. If we can't identify trauma or tragedy as triggers for self-soothing, we will not break cycles of obsession leading to maladjusted behavior.

To build emotional courage, we must penetrate internal layers of denial and shame. We must look at issues related to abandonment, rejection, and betrayal. We must explore past relationships to see if we have given and received love and understanding, attention and affection, as well as kindness, trust, and respect. We must evaluate our capacity for happiness and contentment in the present moment. We must also examine future plans and concerns to deal with the implications of expectation, fear, and anxiety.

Emotions hardly appear without codependent activation or sufficient conditions. When we consider that present feelings may be the effect of past encounters or future projections, we increase our capacity for emotional courage. When we align past and future thoughts within the present moment, emotional discernment and decision-making processes are strengthened. When we establish an authentic view and right speech toward ourselves and others, emotional consistency and decisiveness are the result. When we build emotional courage through honest effort and endure its expansion with boldness, emotional sobriety is imminent.

Below are questions to fortify emotional courage. Read each one slowly and carefully. Pause and reflect on any feelings that arise within you as you internalize these questions. Refrain from self-condemnation or judgment of others. Allow your emotions to naturally expand or contract. Allow your emotional recalibration.

. . .

Why do I drink or use drugs and other substances?

What is the impetus behind my actions that lead to addiction?

When did my harmful or self-defeating behaviors begin?

Was there a specific moment or situation in my life that created a desire to escape reality?

What am I trying to avoid when I succumb to addiction or similar behaviors?

How do I feel about myself today?

Which emotions prevent me from feeling contentment and peace?

Can I release attachment to how I may feel in the future?

Additional options to cultivate emotional courage to consider are therapy, journaling, inner-child healing, and twelve-step work with a sponsor.

MENTAL COURAGE

When stuck in active addiction, many of us may become comfortable with discomfort. We may become accustomed to feelings of low self-esteem and hopelessness because we can't fathom alternate states of being. We may prefer to act from self-pity and tolerate loneliness because at least these are familiar. We may live an uninspired life because we fear the unknown or a change of routine.

Mental courage allows us to abandon old, useless ideas that are not serving our highest good. It gives us space to turn our attention from things like cynicism and sarcasm toward intuitive wisdom. It allows us to avoid procrastination or intolerance so we can become autonomous and focus on efforts to uplift ourselves and others. It allows us to utilize emotional courage so that our decisions and actions can be infused with integrity.

When our thoughts are negative, persistent, and left uncorrected, our intellect will reflect these deficiencies; conversely, when our thoughts are positive and conscious, our perception and presence will reflect these qualities. If we can't repair broken or damaged thought processes, hurtful notions and their corresponding actions will govern our lives. If we can't steer our mentality away from the things that lead to addiction, we will never find recovery.

Mental courage is best strengthened through the process of replacement. When we subtract things that are toxic from our mind, we create space for universal truths, life-affirming ideas, and positive images. When we discard detrimental thoughts, we no longer suffer from indecisiveness, inability to focus, or loss of clarity. When we shed beliefs that are inhibiting our evolution, we can make clear and powerful choices to alter our lives and the lives of those around us.

Below are suggestions to cultivate mental courage. Notice how you concentrate on these tasks. Try to remain in the present moment as you practice these exercises.

Conscious Breathing

Use *ujjayi pranayama*, a yogic-style breathing exercise that can be translated as "victorious or courageous breath." Find a comfortable seat and close your eyes. Gently seal your lips. Inhale and exhale through your nose. Constrict the back of your throat, which will create a subtle, snoring type of sound as the breath moves through this area of the body. Find a steady rhythm for your breath. Focus primarily on the feeling of inhaling and exhaling through your nostrils. Focus next on the sound and sensation being created at the back of your throat. If your mind wanders, bring your awareness back to the breath. Breathe in this style for five minutes, then blink your eyes open. Notice the quality of your mind.

Fruit Meditation

Choose any fruit and find a comfortable, seated position. Hold the fruit in your hands. Look at the colors and shape of the fruit. Feel the texture of the fruit. Bring the fruit to your nose. Notice its fragrance. Realize that sunshine, rain, and soil help fruit to grow. Then close the eyes and imagine the fruit. Call to mind its colors and shape. Remember its texture and fragrance. Contemplate the interdependent relationship between the fruit, sunshine, rain, and soil. Continue to visualize the fruit for a few minutes or until the image naturally fades from your mind. Contemplate how the fruit maintains its integrity and courage to become what it is meant to be despite adverse conditions that may prevent its maturation. Open your eyes when you are finished. Notice if your mind feels concentrated and relaxed. If you are hungry, enjoy your fruit with awareness of how it manifested and with gratitude for its courage to evolve.

Mantra Repetition

Use the yogic mantra *Ong So Hung*, which affirms our oneness with a cosmic consciousness. Find a comfortable position. Pick one spot to look at or close your eyes. Repeat *Ong So Hung* at a pace that feels right to you. Perhaps play a recording of this chant and sing along with it. Allow yourself to believe there is a divine or right and natural order to the universe and you are part of this unfolding process. Allow yourself to believe that your presence is integral to the rhythm of the cosmos. Allow yourself to be inspired by this eternal wisdom. Chant *Ong So Hung* for five minutes, or until you feel that you are finished. Open your eyes if they are closed. When you are done, notice if your mind feels attuned, energized, and stable.

Additional suggestions to cultivate mental courage could be to turn to trusted mentors for support and guidance, to read the works and biographies of inspirational leaders and teachers, to make certain your thoughts are congruent with your words and actions, or to discard prejudice and anything cerebral that does not support a purposeful life.

SPIRITUAL COURAGE

Spiritual courage is stepping into the abyss of uncertainty with extraordinary conviction. It is using the light of inner awareness to guide us through the vicissitudes of life. It is trusting in a higher power or higher purpose and using this belief as a compass to steer ourselves toward a better understanding of life.

Spiritual courage is an assuredness that nearly transcends mortal understanding. It is the ability to have extraordinary faith in something we know to be genuine. It is to inherently perceive that all things are as they are and could not possibly be any other way. It is to believe our lives are precious and useful and that we have always been well and watched over. It is to know we will always be protected and never forsaken.

Spiritual courage is an opportunity to amend what we think we know about ourselves, life, God, spirituality, and our relationships with others. It allows us to conquer personal hesitancy and the impotence of self-will. It helps us overcome the smallness of self and realize we are inextricably connected to all living things. It allows us to look appreciatively in the direction of righteousness and unity rather than bemoan our distance from these destinations.

Spiritual courage inspires us to accomplish tasks that may seem impossible without special assistance. For example, we can forgive those who harm us, remain calm when provoked, leave an abusive relationship, go through a divorce or similar separation, refuse an alcoholic drink in early sobriety, refrain from gossip, speak our innermost truth, pursue higher education, battle cancer, put the welfare of others first, and try to transform our lives in other meaningful ways, including thriving in recovery.

Below are suggestions to cultivate spiritual courage. These practices can be personalized and performed daily or as often and routinely as possible.

Prayer

Prayer strengthens our personal spiritual connection to a God of our own choosing, or any similar holy name or entity that may represent universal strength and protection. Prayer can be offered aloud or in silence; sitting, kneeling, and standing; communicated in solitude or among religious or spiritual friends. Perhaps try the Prayer of St. Francis of Assisi or the Serenity Prayer, or simply and sincerely find a way to ask for what you need. Prayers of gratitude are also powerful.

Yoga

Any style of yoga or sequence of postures will help you connect to your innermost self and stimulate spiritual courage. For example, the standing pose known as *tadasana*, or mountain pose, cultivates solidity and stillness; the sitting pose known as *sukhasana*, or easy pose, allows for discovery of patience and presence; and the supine pose known as *savasana*, or corpse pose, offers the opportunity to learn humility through surrender. Additionally, a dedicated yoga practice integrates and maintains a healthy relationship between emotional, mental, physical, and spiritual forms of courage.

Spiritual Reading

Inspirational reading materials can help you access deeper levels of spiritual awareness and understanding. Dedicate a special time and space for this type of practice. Read for comprehension and view your materials as guides toward inner development. Take notes as you move through your chosen texts. Talk with friends and like-minded seekers about the spiritual topics that interest you. Share your authentic views about your studies and learn to articulate your spiritual beliefs.

Additional suggestions to cultivate spiritual courage could be to read sacred texts and poetry, spend time in nature, listen to guided meditations, sit in silent contemplation, write gratitude lists, enjoy fellowship with spiritually minded peers, or volunteer or participate in service work.

5

Vulnerability

Vulnerability in recovery means to be forthright about personal inadequacies. It is acknowledging our unskillfulness rather than condemning ourselves for simply being human. It means to admit the degree of incongruence and messiness within our lives. It is taking off the proverbial masks we may wear and exposing the blemishes underneath. It is risking embarrassment for the sake of freedom. It is removing any facade built in front of our authenticity so that we can be real, raw, and recovered.

Vulnerability often begins as an alternative or temporary ideal when we leave addiction behind. However, it is hardly something that can be intellectualized or embodied on a part-time basis; it must be adopted as a way of being if it is to lead to emancipation.

When we practice vulnerability, we become sensitized to the unitive state where polarities harmonize. We comprehend the duality of feelings and find equanimity between all seeming opposites. For example, we come to know and respect both the depths of sorrow and heights of joy, the heaviness of hatred and levity of love, the miseries of addiction and miracles of recovery.

To practice vulnerability, we must release personal attachments to the opinions of others. We must become willing to feel weak or appear pathetic. We must find ways to receive ridicule or condemnation with aplomb rather than antagonism. We must become sympathetic toward our own faults and accept all parts of our personality. We must let go of perfectionism.

If we can't integrate vulnerability into our recovery, we will likely withhold secrets that can sicken us or lead to relapse; self-love will be difficult to develop; and feelings of disconnection or loneliness may besiege us.

PRACTICING VULNERABILITY

Vulnerability can be fostered by establishing a solid foundation to support both outward and inward exploration. Additionally, when we investigate the physical and emotional parameters of the *anahata*, or heart chakra, our understanding of vulnerability is deepened.

Below you will find a *kriya*, or dynamic yogic practice, to attain a sense of somatic groundedness and to create spaciousness around the heart. Practitioners can modify this sequence as needed and use variations for the poses and movements to match their level of flexibility. Props can be utilized, such as chairs, blankets, and pillows. And incense or a candle can be lit to help create a sacred practice space.

ONE: Begin in *sukhasana*, or easy pose. Sit cross-legged or in a comfortable, seated position. Root down through your sitting bones. Feel the earth beneath you. Feel a sense of steadiness and belonging. Rest your hands on your knees or in your lap. Take three conscious breaths. Use *ujjayi* breathing, or any preferred method. With each inhale, feel the expansion of your chest. With each exhale, connect to the earth. Relax deeper into your seated pose. Bring your hands together at your heart. Bow your head. Set an intention to know more about vulnerability. Finalize your intention with a deep inhale and exhale.

TWO: Remain seated and place your palms on your knees. Circle the torso from the hips in a clockwise motion. Coordinate your breath and movement. Relax your shoulders and neck. Relax your jaw. Relax your elbows, wrists, and fingers. Relax your knees, ankles, and toes. After a few breaths, change the direction of the circles. Notice where your body may be tense; bring awareness to these areas and release or relax them. Notice the healing benefits of natural movements. When you are ready, discontinue the circles and find stillness.

THREE: Bring your hands together at your heart. Reestablish connection to your seated posture. Feel grounded, steady, and solid. Feel a sense of home and stability. With an inhale, open your arms out wide. With an exhale, bring your hands back together at your heart. Repeat this pattern of expansion/contraction with your next ten breaths. Allow each inhale and exhale to choreograph its corresponding movement. Perhaps close your eyes as you internalize this practice.

FOUR: Lie down on your back in *savasana*, or corpse pose. Rest your arms down by your sides with your palms turned upward. Relax your legs and feet. Remain still. Feel your shoulder blades and the back of your head supported by the earth beneath you. Notice if your heart space feels more open. Close your eyes. Relax in this position for three minutes or longer. Begin to wiggle your fingers and toes. Circle your wrists and ankles. Bring movement back to your body. Reach your arms overhead. Lengthen your spine. Take an inhale and fill your body with breath. Exhale and find peace in the present moment.

FIVE: Gently roll onto the right side of your body into a fetal position. Pause. Recall your intention to know more about vulnerability. Notice if your body feels more energized or stable. Notice if your mind feels more calm or balanced. Notice if your heart feels more open or receptive. Rise to a comfortable, seated position. Bring your hands together at your heart. Lower your chin toward your chest. Thank your body for supporting the practice. Thank your breath, mind, heart, and spirit. Bow to your innermost self to close this practice.

BENEFITS OF VULNERABILITY

When vulnerability works in and through our lives, polarities no longer restrict our perspective. We receive praise and criticism equally. We see all people as teachers. We recognize all experiences as learning moments. We value our defects as assets rather than liabilities. We are no longer emotionally tossed about by what others think or say about our work or character. We are no longer mentally perplexed by how things work. We are not disappointed when the physical body suffers from injury or age. And we do not lack spiritual confidence since vulnerability converts our sufferings and successes into opportunities for growth, connection, and healing.

When we embody vulnerability as a way of being, our mortifications become our message of hope; our mayhem becomes our ministry; and our powerlessness becomes our purpose for living a virtuous life. When vulnerability augments our disposition, our thoughts, words, and actions are forever altered, and our presence gives others encouragement as they journey through recovery. When vulnerability becomes our means for authentic communication and connection in the present moment, a template for all future interactions is created.

THE RECIPROCITY OF VULNERABILITY— A PERSONAL ACCOUNT

When I was sober for six months, I met a young man outside of a twelve-step meeting. He had been sober for only a few days. We stood alone in a parking lot. He wanted to talk about his life and addiction, but he was unable to find the words. He seemed afraid to tell me anything real or honest. I felt a sense of connection with him because I knew what it was to be newly sober. I knew what it felt like to be fearful of telling the truth about anything to anyone. I wanted to help him, but I didn't know how to get him to open up or trust me.

Then I remembered how I had heard other people in recovery share their truth aloud at twelve-step meetings I attended. I remembered how incredible and helpful it had been for me to witness their humility, humanity, and honesty. I remembered how I wanted to someday help others in a similar way.

I realized I could do that now with the young man in front of me. I realized I could give back what I had received. I realized that all I needed to do was be honest about something. I realized that all I needed to do was become vulnerable.

I recalled a secret from my past I had never told to anyone. It was something I figured I would take with me to the grave. But in that moment, I chose instead to be vulnerable and shared my secret with the young man in the parking lot. He listened patiently. Then he shared some things that he needed to talk about. I listened patiently. When he finished, we were both healed.

LET'S MAKE THIS PERSONAL

Read the questions below and become willing to explore the principle of vulnerability in relation to all areas of your life. Contemplate how you can put words to something that you have not yet honestly addressed. Consider writing your responses to these questions in a journal or talking about your processes with a trusted friend who will understand your self-examinations. Remember that vulnerability is a strength and it is essential to recovery.

Is there something that you need to share?

Is there something on your mind that you have not yet told anybody and you feel that now may be the time?

Are you willing to release the burden of trying to remain strong or unaffected by conflicts within your life?

Is there something specific that is blocking you from achieving lasting recovery?

What is keeping you from sobriety?

What prevents you from putting down the bottle? Or putting away the drugs? Or setting aside sugar, caffeine, or nicotine?

What would it take for you to let go of obsessions with the internet, social media, or pornography?

How might you be able to release compulsions toward gambling or shopping?

Whatever your addiction or undesirable behaviors may be, can you open up to the concept of vulnerability in this moment?

Can you share something personal about your life and re-covery, without attachment to how you will be received by others?

How can you practice being vulnerable today?

6

Open-Mindedness

Open-mindedness in recovery is remaining teachable, childlike, curious, and nonjudgmental. It means to be receptive to new concepts, different philosophies, and unfamiliar ideologies. It means a willingness to grow, learn, and evolve rather than stunt our emotional, mental, or spiritual health with patterns of rigidity, stubbornness, or intellectualism.

Many people in recovery can likely admit that when they first got sober, they had specific ideas about what sobriety ought to look like and what they were willing to do to remain sober, clean, or abstinent. And many of them can probably also admit that they needed to expand their views about addiction to find solutions that would bring about lasting recovery.

Consider this prompt often used to help clients in the field of addiction treatment: "We don't know what we don't know."

Now think about these questions: Are you certain that your method to find happiness, peace, or recovery is the right or only way? Are you willing to listen to the viewpoint of another person? Are you sure that you can't learn something beneficial from another source or tradition?

Imagine a room with no door or windows. Imagine the quality of the air in that room. Imagine how dust must collect within it and upon anything inside the room. Imagine the stagnant atmosphere around the perimeter of the room. It is unlikely anything healthy will grow or thrive within a room that is sealed off from outer influence or interaction. Likewise, when the doors and windows of perception within the mind are closed, uninspired beliefs get recycled, thoughts become stale, consciousness is stifled, and the intellect grows malnourished due to a lack of stimulation.

Now imagine another room filled with sunlight, fresh air, and plenty of space. Imagine the room is cleaned often and old or useless things are discarded when they no longer serve an intended purpose. Imagine that new things are added to the room as needed. Imagine the inviting and lively ambience in and around a room that is orderly and uncluttered. Similarly, when the mind is open to new ideas and fresh perspectives, it functions creatively, catalogs our memories and experiences effectively, and underwrites our words and actions harmoniously.

SEEING THINGS FROM A NEW PERSPECTIVE

When the mind is seized by addiction, the scope of what we see narrows and we are unable to view reality clearly; as a result, emotional and mental acuity is unattainable and self-doubt sabotages efforts to find recovery. When our perception is skewed by the kaleidoscopic effects of addiction, self-esteem declines; fear of others cripples us; and feelings of loneliness and separation lead us to dangerous and addictive behaviors. If we can't substitute the lens through which we view the world in active addiction with something else, the aftereffects of such impaired vision can create endless cycles of suffering until the issue can be rectified.

Within the yoga tradition, there is a reliable solution for the misalignment of perspective brought about by addiction. When we utilize the subtle body wisdom of the *chakras,* or wheels of energy within our body, and close the two physical eyes to experience life through the aperture of the *ajna chakra,* or third-eye point, spiritual insight can be developed, which leads to mental recalibration and, naturally, open-mindedness.

The ajna chakra is the command center where intuition, balance, and wisdom reside. Third-eye vision is beyond subjectivity, judgment, and anticipation. From the mystical vantage point of the third eye—slightly above and between the eyebrows—discernment is divine and pragmatic and all sentient things are perceived with impartiality and celebrated with reverence. When we behold the miracles of life through the cognizance of the third-eye portal, joy and wonderment animate consciousness and the mind remains open.

Below are yogic practices to stimulate and harmonize the third-eye center. These exercises develop open-mindedness through self-discipline, concentration, and present-moment awareness.

Mantra Recitation

Aum (or *Om*) is the *bija*, or seed sound, associated with the ajna chakra. When this mantra is repeated with sincerity, *prajna*, or deep insight, is developed, which leads to open-mindedness.

Find a quiet place to sit. Close your eyes. Take your gaze upward to the third eye point between the eyebrows. Inhale to anchor your mind and heart in the present moment. Exhale and recite *Aum* (or *Om*) silently or aloud. Repeat this pattern five times. Pause in stillness and silence. Notice the quality of your mind. Notice if you feel the reverberation and effects of the mantra at the third-eye center.

Asana, or Yoga Pose

Balasana, or child's pose, fortifies third-eye capabilities through physical stimulation as the third eye is set upon the earth within this position.

Find a level or smooth area on the floor or ground. Lay down a yoga mat, towel, or blanket to create a practice space. Come onto your hands and knees. Rest the tops of your feet on the mat. Bring your big toes together behind you. Stretch your hips toward or onto your heels. Stretch your arms forward and set your hands down. Place your third eye on the mat. If your forehead does not rest comfortably on the floor, stack your forearms to create a foundation, or use a pillow or other props for support. Rest in this position for ten breaths. Feel the third eye at rest on the earth. Notice if you feel a sense of groundedness or stability. Notice if you sense humility as you bow down to seek higher knowledge.

Color Visualization Meditation

Indigo is the color associated with the ajna chakra. Imagining this color prepares the third-eye center to clearly reflect reality.

Lie down on your back, or find a comfortable seated position. Bring awareness to the third eye. Bring focus to the concepts of balance, intuition, and wisdom; clarity of thought, speech, and deed; and freedom from the limitations of time and space. Take a conscious in-breath and out-breath. Close your eyes and imagine the color indigo, a shade between blue and violet. Allow this color to fill the landscape of your mind. Breathe deeply and slowly ten times. Continue to visualize the color indigo. Remain open to seeing other colors and images that may arise within your mind as well. When you are ready, open your eyes. Notice the tone of the colors around you. Notice if there is a sense of lucidity within your mind, a feeling of grace within your heart, or an awareness of unity within your spirit or soul.

LET'S MAKE THIS PERSONAL

When the mind remains open, the heart becomes attuned accordingly and radiates empathy, compassion, and understanding into the world through our words and actions. When both the mind and heart are open, we possess clarity and strength to accomplish that which otherwise challenges our resolve, such as forgive long-standing grievances, become truly selfless, and persevere through periods of confusion or darkness. When we become open-minded and openhearted, our collective purpose to awaken to an individual calling may be fulfilled and we know how to do what needs to be done and do it as best as we can.

Read and contemplate the questions below. Discuss your answers with a friend in recovery or another person you can trust. Perhaps write down your reflections in a diary. Remember that open-mindedness leads to openheartedness, and both these qualities are necessary to sustain recovery.

How can you be more open-minded today?

Are you willing to set aside certain beliefs or conceptual limitations to view all people, places, and things as learning experiences or teaching moments?

Are you willing to learn from nature or the elements? For example, can you learn solidity from mountains? Fluidity from rivers? Freshness and beauty from flowers? Alchemy from fire? Impermanence from the leaves on your favorite tree?

Can you learn from birds in the air to see things from a higher perspective? Can you learn impermanence from clouds in the sky? Can you learn about interdependence from all the things around you?

What can you discover about yourself and life from your experiences with things like anxiety, fear, shame, or despair?

Would you be willing to view addiction as one of your greatest teachers?

Can you name five positive things that your recovery has recently revealed to you?

Can you be more open-minded in regard to your current views about spirituality or mindfulness?

Can you be more accepting of the struggles and needs of others?

Are you willing to allow your heart to open fully? What are you willing to do so that this can happen?

How can you express openheartedness to yourself and to those in need today?

7

Consistency

Consistency in recovery means to have a routine. It is adhering to habitual practices that generate positive effects. It is offering undivided attention to that which has been prioritized as noteworthy and transformative. It means to employ repetitiveness and reinforcement to create harmony within the territories of the mind, body, and spirit in order to uplift our thoughts, words, and actions.

For many people in recovery, consistency may begin as an effort to steer our lives toward a particular destination. However, when beneficial disciplines are repeated with diligence and self-sacrifice, notions that may have seemed dull or theoretical can become joyful and embodied; eagerness replaces apathy as we accomplish tasks to alter our consciousness and we no longer need to try to get or stay sober but become and remain sober as a result of dedication.

When we devote time and energy to specific, transcendent exercises, an intuitive wisdom or higher intelligence carries our endeavors to fruition. When we continue to show up for ourselves in this manner, divine guidance becomes a teacher in all areas of our lives. When we remain resilient through purposeful action, consistency removes the doer from the doing; effort becomes effortless; and we transcend sickness and indolence to achieve health and freedom.

Most people in recovery are already familiar with consistency. For example, we may regularly attend twelve-step or similar meetings, talk often with a sponsor or therapist, and try to help newcomers whenever possible. Contrarily, within active addiction, we may have continually engaged in self-destructive behaviors, purposely avoided self-care, and perpetuated a detrimental standard of living. If consistency contributes to a better quality of life whether we remain sober or not, we ought to consciously choose how to practice this principle so we can live in an orderly and purposeful way.

PRACTICING CONSISTENCY

Within the yoga tradition, the concept of *sadhana*, which can be defined as "daily practice," provides a template for how to be consistent and create a framework to maintain recovery. A sadhana honors specific rituals or teachings that lead to a desired, ultimate goal by enthusiastically focusing on the work at hand, renouncing all things that don't enrich the path toward the goal, and relinquishing selfish attachments for the attainment of the goal. Additionally, a sadhana can deliver seekers an awareness of the presence of God, the divine nature within all things, and similar expressions of unification, enlightenment, and emancipation.

A sadhana can be personally curated to suit the needs, skills, resources, and goals of each student or seeker. To create a sadhana, a person can first choose a precise objective. Next, practices that lead toward that objective can be selected. Last, steadiness, reverence, and humility can be guiding principles as a sadhana is observed.

Below are suggestions for things people in recovery can do to create a personal sadhana. Try these or similar methods to customize a daily practice that works best for you.

Prayer

Use prayers or other contemplations that resonate with your beliefs and lifestyle. Petition to a God or higher power of your own understanding. Popular prayers in recovery include the Serenity Prayer, the Lord's Prayer, and the Prayer of St. Francis of Assisi. Prayers of gratitude can also be helpful, as well as prayers to enhance the lives of others.

Meditation

Choose a style of meditation that you prefer. Find a comfortable position so that your experience is enjoyable. Create a sacred space within your home for your practice, or choose a safe and quiet space outdoors. Common meditation methods include conscious breathing, scanning the body with mindfulness, and visualization techniques.

Journaling

Use a notebook or some other means to record your thoughts. Detail and process the events within your day. Catalog your feelings, observations, and memories. Perhaps write a gratitude list, compose poems, or create artwork.

Reading

Select an inspirational book and study its chapters or passages. Sit somewhere quiet and private to contemplate the meaning of the material. Keep paper and pen nearby to take notes.

Conscious Movement

Strengthen your body with yoga, walking, tai chi, qigong, dance, and similar disciplines. Attend group classes at a local studio or community center. Watch video tutorials for inspiration. Choreograph your own sessions or workouts and practice at home or in nature.

Note: For maximum benefit, be intentional with how and when you perform your sadhana. For example, you can practice prayer and meditation each morning; write in a journal each afternoon; read and utilize conscious movement every evening. As personal tastes and practices evolve over time, be willing to adapt and revitalize your sadhana as needed.

LET'S MAKE THIS PERSONAL

To discover and improve your current consistency habits, take an inventory of what you do on a daily basis. First, make a list of favorable things you do for yourself each day. For example, many people can recognize that they consistently brush their teeth, eat, exercise, and bathe or shower.

Next, make a list of things you do for yourself each day that may not serve a higher purpose. For example, many people may recognize that they squander time reading certain magazines, watching specific programs on TV, and browsing particular websites on the internet.

Then look at your lists. Can you recognize patterns? Where and how do you spend your time and energy? Do your daily activities lead you toward or away from happiness, contentment, and recovery? Where can you make adjustments or choose different things to do? Where can you replace certain behaviors with things better suited for a life you feel called to live in recovery?

Within recovery, there is a phrase to help people find balance within their lives: "The way we do anything is the way we do everything." If the things on our lists are not aligned with the principles we wish to practice in recovery, we ought to notice where changes can be made so that consistency regulates our life and all our endeavors lead to liberation, joy, and peace.

CREATING AND MAINTAINING POSITIVE CONSISTENCY HABITS

Lasting recovery is hardly something we can achieve through luck or half-hearted effort. Some people may find short-term sobriety with these types of approaches; however, if long-term recovery is our goal, consistency is essential. We must find methods to continuously do things that help us remain healthy at the levels of mind, body, and spirit. We must commit to plans of action each day that support the maturation of our recovery. And we must integrate insights obtained within daily practices into all our affairs.

When we are consistent with how we nourish the mind, body, and spirit, we learn to love and trust ourselves, and others come to depend upon our reliability and fortitude. When we do positive things in a systematic manner, our self-confidence increases and irritations can be accepted as opportunities to realize new levels of freedom. When consistency anchors our days, our character becomes appropriately molded, and successes in recovery and life can be attributed to sustained effort.

Below are suggestions that can augment our aptitude to remain consistent. Modify these activities as needed. Practice individually or alongside friends in recovery.

Choose a beneficial habit or activity you are interested in learning more about and do it consecutively for seven days. At the end of this time frame, assess what you have learned and share your experience with someone who can offer an objective interpretation about your progress.

Organize a specialized weekly meeting for others in recovery. Gather artists, single parents, cancer survivors, or any group of people who share a common issue or interest. Choose when the group will meet and structure each gathering so every member can feel welcome.

Join a book study group and regularly interact with other participants through public or private forums to discuss your interpretations of the subject matter.

Register for a weekly or monthly volunteer shift at a local shelter, food bank, or nursing home.

Participate in a thirty-day yoga or meditation challenge at a neighborhood studio or online.

If you attend twelve-step or other recovery-based meetings, attend thirty meetings in thirty days. Additionally, take a service commitment at one of these meetings.

Chant your favorite yogic mantra or recite a positive affirmation 108 times each day for a week. You can use a mala bead necklace and count each of its 108 beads as you recite your chant or look into a mirror and offer your phrase to the highest good within you as you honor your reflection.

8

Transparency

Transparency in recovery is centered on being forthright and honest no matter the cost. It is setting aside attachment to personal reputation in honor of the truth. It means saying and doing what is right despite fear or embarrassment and trusting that this process purifies the soul. It is a type of housekeeping to rid the mind, body, and spirit of that which leads to addictions.

Without transparency in recovery, we may find ourselves living in a state of ambiguity. We may eschew facts so that detrimental habits and unhealthy interactions become bearable. We may be unable to distinguish significant or irrelevant memories and moments. We may lie about things, real or imagined, to feel a sense of normalcy. We may come to realize vagueness not only masks truths but casts shadows over the entirety of our lives.

Additionally, if transparency is not observed in recovery, our intentions will become unclear and we will squander our time and vitality. Our ethical code will be impaired, and we may find ourselves defending personal narratives that serve lower energies. Our willpower and motivation will decline, and we will become susceptible to desires or cravings for alcohol, drugs, and other substances.

Addiction feeds on those who are indecisive, cynical, or opaque with their thought processes. It targets those detached from truth, abducts the integrity of those who are self-involved, and preys on those with low self-esteem. It assails all people who are disconnected from morality and overwhelms anyone who indulges philosophies of self-hatred.

Transparency begets self-respect, without which the sanctity of recovery remains unprotected from attacks dispatched by addiction. If we can't grasp the importance of transparency and purify our emotional, mental, intellectual, physical, and spiritual health, lasting recovery may not be possible. Transparency is hardly optional for those in recovery; it is essential if we wish to know serenity and sovereignty.

Ultimately, transparency in recovery allows us to maintain purpose and clarity as it removes shallow or false stories placed ahead of the actuality of our existence. It gives us permission to no longer be deceptive as adherence to its tenets expunges impulses to alter reality. It prompts us to ask ourselves what we are hiding and why. It grants us the gifts of lucidity and genuineness as it guides us toward inmost truths. It invites us to be intentional with how we move about the world. It is indeed the gauge by which we assess the purity of recovery.

BECOMING TRANSPARENT

Within the Yoga Sutras of Patanjali, the concept of *saucha*, which is presented as a self-discipline for cleanliness, exemplifies how to be transparent. Saucha is a process of purification. It is to be selective and strict with what we allow to enter and remain within the mind, body, and spirit. It can also be viewed as a form of detoxification by which the intellect becomes luminescent.

When saucha is observed, qualities that no longer serve a higher purpose, such as deceitfulness, immorality, vanity, and other deficiencies, may be removed from our consciousness. Saucha refines our perception, an improvement that eliminates fear, guilt, and remorse from our thoughts, speech, and actions. When our mentality is cleansed and upgraded in these ways, inherent qualities such as love, compassion, and understanding oversee our personal and worldly affairs.

Both saucha and recovery address the necessity for transparency within the mind, body, and spirit. These three realms are independent yet interdependent; therefore, all must remain pure and unified for optimum health. Below are prompts to examine how we nourish the mind, body, and spirit and suggestions to harmonize these areas so that transparency can properly influence our recovery and all our affairs.

Mind

What holds space within your thought forms? What do you think about most often? Where do your thoughts travel throughout the day? What do you dream about? What are your goals? What do you aspire to achieve? What are your priorities? Are you harboring secrets, resentments, or fears? How do you renew your mind? Do you take part in conversations or interactions that include gossip, sarcasm, or discrimination? Do you set meaningful intentions? What types of things do you listen to, watch, or read?

If aspects of the mind are impure or unbalanced, make specific choices to neutralize and transform these things. If there is something you need to tell someone to clear your conscience, find someone you trust and talk to them. If you are not pursuing your purpose, redirect your efforts to align yourself with an inner calling. If you continue to indulge harmful, limiting beliefs, seek help to change these patterns. If you are feeding the mind toxins in any form, cease these types of behavior and choose positive alternatives.

Body

How do you honor your body? Do you eat nutritious foods in appropriate amounts? Do you know where your food comes from? Do you bathe and shower regularly? Do you care for your skin? Do you wash your clothes often? Do you care for your teeth? Is your home clean and free of clutter? Do you visit medical and therapeutic professionals as necessary? Do you exercise? Are certain areas of your body tense or tight? How is your breathing? How is the health of your heart?

If you eat food that lacks sustenance, alter or supplement your diet to receive proper nutriments. If you remain stationary throughout the day, take regular walks or practice yoga to increase blood flow in the body. If you are irregular with hygiene habits, adhere to a schedule so the body remains free from inner impurities and outer contaminants. If your home or work surroundings are chaotic, organize your affairs and eliminate distractions. If you take part in activities that dishonor your body or the bodies of others, examine your motives and redirect your energies toward wholesome endeavors.

Spirit

What does spirituality mean to you? How do you connect to God or divinity in its many forms? Do you pray or meditate? Do you spend time in nature? Are you able to find gratitude for your life? Can you connect to your innermost self? Can you be at peace when you are alone? Do you use spiritual books or other inspirational materials for daily practices? What are your self-care rituals? Do you have spiritual fellowship with like-minded peers or friends in recovery?

If your own strength does not solve your problems, seek guidance and help from a higher perspective. If your mind is cloudy or your heart is closed, meditate on expressions of purity and openness. If your intentions are unclear, think of God, Nature, Mother Earth, and similar conceptions that represent an ultimate truth or absolute reality. If you feel lonely, imagine things that reflect the unity or oneness of life. If you feel depressed, draw upon the power of prayer to illuminate your spirit. If you feel anxiety, cultivate gratitude for opportunities to grow and learn. If your life lacks meaning, offer your time, energy, and resources in service to others.

BENEFITS OF TRANSPARENCY

Just as a clear prism receives and refracts light to expose natural colors, when we embrace transparency, intrinsic principles such as empathy, kindness, and brotherhood manifest. When a prism is unlit or blemished, colors can't appear; similarly, without transparency as part of recovery, psychological darkness permeates our consciousness.

When we are transparent in recovery, self-absorption is replaced by a worldview based on neutrality. We lose a separate sense of self and are no longer limited by ideas of duality or affected by opinions of others. We no longer suffer from bewilderment as our thoughts, words, and actions become aligned. We no longer fear incidents from the past nor concerns about the future. And we have nothing to hide as we become fully available and alive in the present moment.

9

Accountability

Accountability is a commonplace and expected manifestation of right or civil conduct within many areas of life. For example, employees are accountable to an employer or supervisor and coworkers; people who live in well-populated areas are accountable to neighbors, law enforcement personnel, and those who hold state and city agency positions; and husbands, wives, and those in similar partnerships are accountable to their spouse and other family members.

For people in recovery, however, accountability determines if we are to know sickness or health, smallness or magnanimity, even life or death. If accountability is missing from the lives of people in recovery, feelings of contentment, purposefulness, and self-confidence will be too; a sense of safety or belonging won't be established; and trust within relationships can't be maintained.

Without accountability in recovery, our thoughts and actions are left unchecked by a supportive, unbiased, or objective perspective, which is just asking for ego inflation. When we become the sole arbiters of our endeavors, we may regress into harmful behaviors and find ourselves without a lifeline if we morally backslide. Such degradation may bring loss of employment, exclusion from community, and deterioration of family relations, among other problems.

When alcoholism or addiction has wreaked havoc in our lives, it is imperative that accountability guides our conscience in recovery, or self-pride will direct our choices and rigidity will be the result. When areas of our lives remain enigmatic, selfish motives will overtake our consciousness, and we will become defensive and abrasive when confronted by things that do not align with our perspective. When we deny individual, collective, or spiritual culpability, anger will command our temperament, and we will utilize justifications and untruths to distance ourselves from our obligations, occupations, and societal duties.

Accountability is indispensable for individuals in recovery and must guide our inner thoughts and outer dealings. If we are not accountable in recovery, we will be assailed by fears, doubts, and anger; jealousy, discrimination, and enmity; lethargy and procrastination. If we do not prioritize accountability within recovery, shame and regret will overshadow our lives; we will become susceptible to deceitfulness, which will engender low self-worth; and we will not experience fidelity within our relationships.

Accountability in recovery begins with self-discipline and how we honor ourselves. Then we look outward at how we regard and relate to others in recovery. Last, we determine how we pursue connection with God or a higher perspective and how our life and recovery reflect this union. Below are suggestions to generate accountability within these three areas and corresponding yogic concepts and practices to stimulate awareness and integration of these ideas.

ACCOUNTABILITY TO ONESELF

We honor our intuition. We say what we feel called to say and we tell the truth. We follow through when we make commitments. We take part in activities that uplift our consciousness. We eat foods that nourish and energize the body. We exercise to keep the body strong and agile. We establish balance between rest and recreation. We commune with nature. We commit to living our best life each day.

The yogic practice of *atma vichara*, or self-inquiry, helps us become conscientious about how we adhere to personal moral codes and self-disciplines. It means returning home to the innermost self and surveying the mind and heart to affirm if beliefs and intentions are aligned and consistent with words and actions. It is how we ascertain if our behavior is congruent with everlasting values.

Atma vichara can be practiced through journaling, meditation, and similar modes of introspection. Ask yourself the following questions and write about your answers, or use these considerations as prompts to guide meditation: Did I do what I set out to do today? Was I honest with myself about my feelings or emotions? Was I kind to my mind, body, and spirit? Did I speak and act with integrity? Did I preserve healthy boundaries and live within my means? Is there anything I need to process or release? Is there something I need to talk about with someone else?

ACCOUNTABILITY TO OTHERS

We tell others what is happening in our lives, and we know what is happening in their lives. We keep promises if we make them. We offer our time and energy if we can be of service. We maintain cleanliness and decorum where we live and work. We honor moral obligations and pay financial debts. We share material and spiritual resources. We uplift those in need and accept encouragement from others. We exemplify hopefulness and vitality through all our interactions.

The Sanskrit term *kalyana mitra* can be defined as "spiritual companions." It means a group of like-minded friends with whom we share truths and concerns. It is people we trust, whose suggestions and solutions are appreciated and reciprocated. It is a collection of seekers bonded through common goals and interests who interrelate with openness, compassion, and equality, as well as dedication, trustfulness, and confidentiality.

Examples of kalyana mitra can be found within twelve-step traditions as fellowships of people gathering with sponsors and other members to share experience, strength, and hope; within Buddhist traditions as *sanghas*, or communities, assembling with monks, nuns, and lay practitioners for meditation, recitation of precepts, and similar disciplines; and within yoga collectives as *kulas*, or groups comprising of teachers, students, and like-minded peers practicing yoga, chanting, and performing *seva*, or selfless acts of service.

Ask yourself the following questions to incorporate the power of kinship into your life and recovery: Who is part of my inner circle? Do I have people in my life that I can trust? Where can I say things I need to say without fear of judgment or ridicule?

Who offers me helpful suggestions? Am I able to listen to others when they need to unburden what is in their hearts? Do I give undivided attention and unbiased affection to friends in need?

If you don't have sober friends or companions in recovery with whom you entrust all aspects of your life, consider joining a recovery-themed group that meets each week. You can also organize a similarly themed gathering for yourself and others based on shared interests or occupations.

ACCOUNTABILITY TO GOD

We dedicate time to prayer and meditation. We ask for divine guidance throughout the day. We offer our energy and resources in service to a higher or spiritual purpose. We align our thoughts, words, and actions in ways that are beneficial and benevolent toward all living beings. We seek to deepen our relationship with what we choose to call God or a higher power. We recognize the spark and source of divinity within all beings. We use the life we have been given to in turn give and receive love.

Within the Yoga Sutras of Patanjali, the moral code of *brahmacharya* is presented as a guide for how to live a sacred life. *Brahmacharya* can be translated as "walking with God." It is viewed as moderation of the senses, which protects and preserves our *prana*, or life force. It is to do what is right, divine, and orderly so that we can leave behind ephemeral sensory pleasures and attain everlasting joy and contentment. It means to remain steady on a personal path of sanctity so that we can align human consciousness with higher awareness and personal willfulness with divine direction.

Examples of how to live a virtuous life are available across various traditions: Moses brought the Ten Commandments to his people; Jesus offered the Eight Beatitudes in his Sermon on the Mount; the Buddha shared the Four Noble Truths and his subsequent Eightfold Path; and Patanjali outlined the *yamas* and *nimayas*, a set of ten universal principles—within which brahmacharya is found—in the Yoga Sutras.

To practice brahmacharya and to establish accountability with God, imagine if you were to ask God or your higher power for permission before doing something that could be considered immoral, illegal, or unsafe. Imagine if you were to seek the approval of God or blessings from an omnipotent and omniscient authority before acting in ways that could undermine your propriety or jeopardize your recovery. Imagine if your conception of God would support all your proposals.

Additionally, consider these questions throughout the day: How have I properly used my inherent talents or skills? Where have I offered love? Have I forgiven others? Whom have I comforted or helped without attachment to reward or recognition? Have I been able to deny selfishness and take contrary action toward a greater or collective good? What can I be grateful for? Can I recognize the place within me where I connect to God and all sentient things? Can I appreciate the miracle of life?

Note: For those who may not have a personal God, an acronym used within the field of addiction recovery may be helpful: G.O.D. = Good Orderly Direction. Consider this substitution to elevate your thoughts and actions in accordance with what may generally be considered inspirational, accurate, and honorable.

ADVANTAGES OF ACCOUNTABILITY

The benefits of accountability for people in recovery are undeniable, immeasurable, and accrue through practice and interaction with others in society. The following are examples of how accountability manifests within the lives of those who make every effort to comprehend its facets, applications, and effects: Acquisition of forthrightness and integrity when we acknowledge our limitations and ask for assistance. Eradication of shame and judgment from the mind and heart when we share passions or goals, admit faults or mistakes, or articulate difficult emotions and experiences. Comprehension of equality when we become part of a community within which all members are integral parts of the whole. Increased humility and openheartedness when we are entrusted to be a safe haven for others and are willing to receive similar support. Attainment of unity and harmony when we no longer remain isolated or self-involved. And reciprocal growth and maturation when our hearts become mirrors for the hearts of others through moral reassurance and soul reinforcement.

10

Perseverance

Perseverance is an ability to endure challenges or setbacks in order to achieve a goal. It is a means by which victory can be guaranteed over internal weaknesses such as procrastination, laziness, and self-centeredness. It propels us toward and through situations we might otherwise avoid due to lack of confidence, fear of failure, and anticipation of judgment or ridicule.

Imagine a long-distance race or similar competition. Athletes invest time, energy, money, and additional resources to methodize strategies in order to win. They endure exhaustion, self-doubt, impatience, and other personal conditions that stand before success. They overcome hostile rivalries and harsh environmental factors to reach their destination. These are examples of how perseverance provides emotional sustenance, mental motivation, and physical stamina on the way to a literal finish line.

Perseverance in recovery, however, means moving with as much, if not more, resolve toward a figurative finish line. It is to advance without knowledge of what lies ahead, to do the next right thing when results can't be foreseen, to know in our hearts that we will be guided and unharmed even if our pace is uneven and the path ahead is unpredictable. It is acquiring spiritual awareness through faithfulness and persistence.

Perseverance in recovery provides wins over weaknesses, triumphs over temptations, and conquests over controversies when it underscores our thoughts, words, and actions. It replaces weariness with enthusiasm when we commit to advancement regardless of egocentric troubles or worldly distractions. It assures contentment when we focus on commencements and continuousness rather than contentiousness or completions.

THOUGHTS, ACTIONS, AND PERSEVERANCE

Perseverance in recovery proceeds through positive action. It is focusing on and performing one thing at a time without attachment to the results of our activities. It means to be conscientious about how we think, speak, and act and regulate our thoughts, words, and deeds in accordance with higher ideals.

To practice perseverance in recovery, we must first examine our personal thoughts that inform consequent actions. We must discern if our intentions are pure and affiliated with wholesome values. We must discover if our driving desires are noble or if ulterior motives are influencing our conscience. We must also assess our daily routines and purge negative influences that inhibit positive thought, speech, and action.

When we understand that thought precedes action, we will realize active addiction often results from negative premeditation. For example, the thought to open a bottle of alcohol comes before we drink; the thought to call the drug dealer comes before we use; the thought to visit the casino comes before we gamble; the thought to act out sexually comes before these behaviors; and additional thoughts to remove ourselves from the present moment or attempt to alter reality come before we engage in such self-deceptive patterns.

When we monitor the mind and replace thoughts that breed negativity with positive concepts, our actions become profitable and the quality of our recovery rises. When we become mindful about how we think and act, our intellectual power increases and spiritual prosperity is acquired. When right thinking and right action become habitual, ideas that lead to addiction become worthless, and perseverance secures its place as the backbone of our recovery.

PRACTICING PERSEVERANCE

Within the yoga tradition, *karma* is defined as action. It also describes things that are done and how they are accomplished; a cause-and-effect type of relationship that affects all areas of life; and the sum of past actions that have created our present circumstances, which in turn, foretell our future.

There is a saying within yogic circles: "The karma meter is always on." Therefore, our day-to-day thoughts, words, and actions determine the quality of our lives. How we think about

phenomena, how we speak to others, how we act in public or behind closed doors—all these things are accounted for and create
innumerable results.

For those in recovery, karma can be considered a cosmic
judicial system activated by a personal willingness or reluctance
to continuously act in harmony with spiritual principles. For
example, if an alcoholic drinks every night, they may experience a hangover each morning, then lie to supervisors to avoid
work, and eventually lose their job due to truancy as the pattern continues. If a gambler spends all their money, they may
get handed an eviction notice when they can't pay rent, then
steal money from others to make ends meet, and may be caught
by police and arrested. And if a sex addict can't stop their behavior, they may contract and spread disease, then suffer from
humiliation and fearfulness, and if the cycle continues, their
spouse or partner may discover their unfaithfulness and offer
them the choice of treatment or demand a divorce or separation.

Karma is impersonal. It can't be purchased or hoodwinked.
It does not care if we are rich or poor, old or young, educated
or unlearned. It does not attack nor take pity on anyone. It is
nondiscriminatory; its rewards are meted out uniformly and
equitably as they are enacted personally and collectively. However, the laws of karma assure us that those who consciously
shape their lives along right lines receive right results, and those
who think, speak, and act with abandon suffer the consequences
of their choices.

Consider the following suggestions to nurture soundness of
mind in order to generate strategic action so that the principle of
perseverance will be integrated with the laws of karma:

. . .

Practice yoga every day for a week. Take classes at a local studio, utilize a live broadcast, or play a prerecorded video.

Call three people in recovery each day for ten consecutive days and ask them about their recovery. Call one person with more time sober than you, another person who has been sober the same length of time as you, and someone else who has less time sober than you.

Meditate for twenty-one days in a row. Use recorded, guided meditations to assist your practice or attend in-person sessions with a teacher and other students. You can also sit and meditate in solitude within your home or at another quiet location.

Write down thirty things that you are grateful for each evening for a month. Keep these pages together in a folder or notebook. At the end of the month, share your causes for gratitude with a mentor or friends in recovery.

Attend fifty twelve-step or similarly themed meetings in fifty days. At the end of this period, assess how you feel and perhaps commit to another set of meetings.

LET'S MAKE THIS PERSONAL

Perseverance in recovery is not a theory to be contemplated. It is not a transitory or intellectual mechanism utilized to obtain specific things. It is action in harmony. Similarly, karma and its ramifications can't be ignored, rationalized, or doubted. It must be viewed as a vehicle for moral regulation and spiritual development.

When we internalize these concepts, we will notice that intentional thoughts, words, and actions transform wayward inner energies, revolutionize our sense of self, and illumine the soul. We will realize we have free will to choose how we react to inner and outer stimuli and that our choices affect all facets of our lives. We can then shape our destiny with deliberate choices and actions that not only improve the quality of our lives but also impact our contribution to humanity.

When we persevere through all situations and our actions emanate from a purified mentality, false narratives within the mind are rewritten to reflect our true valor; destructive compulsions are forever quelled; and our overall health is restored to optimum levels. When we exhibit toughness and endurance in the face of addiction and other forms of suffering, our disposition is forever altered and our capacity to withstand trials and adversities on our path toward wellness is solidified. When our consciousness is shielded by perseverance and our actions originate from a lucid mind, apathy and cowardice become foreign to us, and we no longer entertain whims or desires to return to old default behaviors.

Use the following questions to reveal where the benefits of perseverance can affect your life and how your thoughts and actions determine the quality of your recovery.

How do you nourish your thoughts? What are your thoughts today about recovery? Can you recognize where your thoughts have preceded certain actions?

What are some positive actions you have taken this week to ensure your sobriety? Is your conduct consistent? Do you have a daily routine to maintain the quality of your recovery?

Have you recently succumbed to or surmounted moments of laziness or selfishness? How do you manage your time? Where in your life do you consistently practice perseverance to support your recovery?

What things will you do today that will affect your future? For example: How will you nourish your body? How will you work? How will you talk with your elders, friends, children, coworkers, neighbors? Where will you be helpful? How will you live your life when no one is watching? Will you be generous with your presence, resources, and love?

How do you know what to do in recovery? Which people or what do you turn to for advice or suggestions? Where do you receive encouragement and how often?

What do you do when your energy is depleted or your spirit is weak? How do you move forward when you feel like giving up or quitting? How do you replenish yourself?

Meditate on your reactions to these questions. Share your answers with someone you trust. Remember that change in recovery is gradual. Remember that awareness of how we think and act is the key to perseverance. Remember that transformation is hardly an overnight matter, yet through recognition of personal issues and proper redirection of our energies, we can alter our experiences, enhance our recovery, and enrich our lives one thought and one action and one day at a time.

11

Punctuality

Punctuality is acknowledging and respecting your own personal time and the time of others. It means adhering to commonly recognized schedules and agreements. It is moving about the world in a consistent and logical manner.

When we think about punctuality, linear time is typically the gauge by which a person or thing is deemed punctual. For example, if we are supposed to start work at 9 a.m. each morning, we arrive at our workplace at this time. If we wish to watch a television program that is broadcast at 2 p.m. every day, we turn on the TV at that time. If we are going to attend a twelve-step meeting, we can presume it begins and ends as listed in a directory. If we bring friends to the airport, we drop them off before their plane departs. If we go to a movie theater, we expect films to start and finish as advertised. If we buy tickets for concerts, plays, recitals, and similar performances, we trust these events will commence at the time advertised. If we make appointments with a doctor or dentist, we presume these plans will be honored. If we want to take a yoga class, we will get to the studio before the teacher begins their instruction. And if we attend religious or spiritual gatherings, the services are likely to begin at the right moment in time as expected.

When punctuality and linear time are individually and collectively observed in all departments of life, protocols are defined and etiquette is established. When our lives become organized in accordance with such established rules, customs, and behaviors, we come to know the meaning of order, structure, and stability. When we acknowledge the value of chronology and accept the certainties and patterns of its facets, our conformity contributes to a communal sense of equivalence, surety, and harmony.

The need for punctuality can be proven by the proliferation of instruments available to measure time—watches, clocks, alarms, timers, and calendars. However, the urgency of punctuality for people in recovery can be more difficult to pin down, as there are no devices to quantify what is unknown or ethereal.

The ancient Greeks used two terms for time: *chronos*, which refers to linear time, and *kairos*, which indicates divine time. The former is sequential and straightforward, as outlined in the examples above. For those in recovery, however, if the latter can't be assessed and cultivated, opportunities to utilize or appreciate the former may be lacking.

DIVINE TIME

Within yogic philosophy, the term *brahma muhurta* can be defined as "divine time" or "time of the gods." It refers to an approximately ninety-minute period before the sun rises each morning. During this predawn interval, our consciousness has not yet been influenced by sounds or movements of the imminent day; therefore, the mind is tranquil, the heart is open, and the veil between earthly and heavenly realms is transparent.

When we utilize this auspicious time for meditation and spiritual practices, we journey inward toward the *anandamaya kosha*, or bliss sheath at the center of our being, where mysteries of eternity are intuited and our *svadharma*, or personal purpose in life, is revealed and understood. During this sojourn, there are no schedules to keep nor any need for haste; there are no barriers to spiritual growth nor limitations to evolutionary development. When we negotiate this inner expedition, we transcend the confinements of linear time and become acquainted with timelessness.

Quietude, serenity, and a sense of the oneness among all sentient things are the hallmarks of timelessness. When we access this state of prescience, we are emancipated from the grip of sequentiality and freed from the minutiae of seconds, minutes, hours, months, and years. We become acquainted with an incomparable sense of spaciousness, and the mind and body attune to the *ritam*, or rhythm of the cosmos. We embrace stillness and silence, and our temperament is recalibrated to comprehend intuitive thoughts. When we apply what is gleaned from these experiences to the material plane of existence, including all areas of recovery, we become efficient, succinct, and punctual.

Spiritual maturation can't be evaluated by chronological time.

Likewise, spiritual solutions to human problems can't be sourced amid mortal chaos. If we wish to rise above addiction, depression, grief, and similar conditions, we must enter the inmost world by means of sacred wandering and explore transcendental moments. We must transmute our awareness of time through meditation and related disciplines that encourage introspection. We must familiarize ourselves with the luminosity of our interiority if we are to know the rewards of punctuality, which include self-esteem, respectability, and purposefulness.

LET'S MAKE THIS PERSONAL

What is your relationship with time? Are there areas of your life where you are stalling? Where you are being lazy? Where you are procrastinating? In which areas of your life are you habitually late?

What keeps you from showing up for yourself on time? Have you had ideas or thoughts that once seemed useful, but you have not acted on them yet? What is holding you back from being punctual? Do you fear judgment or ridicule? Do you fear failure or success? Does perfectionism render you immobile?

If you are not yet sober but want to be, is now the time to do it? If not now—when? What are you waiting for?

If you are already in recovery, are there things you feel called to do but you have not done them yet? Is now the time? If not now—when? What are you waiting for?

Do you make excuses for your lack of action or tardiness? Which feelings or emotions arise in you when you are late? How do you feel about yourself when you postpone important things? How do you feel about yourself when you are punctual?

Is it time for you to grow up or become more mature? To talk to your partner about something within your relationship? To consider another career path or look for another job? To work on issues that are keeping you from being your best self?

Is it time for you to put away a grudge? To make amends? To forgive someone? To figure out why you are lonely, angry, or depressed? To ask for help or offer assistance to someone else in need? To speak your truth at home or work? To open your heart?

Are you willing to believe there is a divine order to life? A sacred manner by which things are arranged for you and all living beings? Are you willing to set aside prejudice to embrace a spiritual life that may be waiting for you?

Are you willing to explore the parameters of timelessness? To cultivate stillness and silence and look within yourself to see and feel things that can help you make good use of linear time? Are you willing to dedicate yourself to practices that create and support calmness and self-reflection so that you can ascertain what may be beneficial, purposeful, or providential in your life?

PRACTICING PUNCTUALITY

Addiction is a predator and thief. It stalks its prey and steals many treasures from its victims, including innocence, morality, and intelligence. However, the most valuable thing it pilfers from unsuspecting people who are slaves to compulsive patterns and behaviors is time. When addiction seizes our days, weeks, years, and decades, we can never reclaim these moments. When time is ripped from our lives by addiction, it is gone forever.

Our best defense to preserve and protect the gift of time from the clutches of addiction is an awareness of punctuality. When we live fully and deeply in the present moment, autonomy is the reward, and we remain custodians of our own choices and agendas. When we are prudent with how we think about and utilize time, we learn to maximize our moments rather than squander them in ways that do not benefit our highest good. When we consider time an unrenewable, priceless commodity, we realize life is a miracle and cherish our path to recovery.

Below are suggestions to further explore a relationship with punctuality and conceptions of time and timelessness.

Punctuality

Explore what steps you can take to arrive early to meetings and other engagements. Plan ahead for traffic, interruptions, and unpredictable factors that can create anxiety and tardiness. Set alarms and reminders on appropriate devices so you don't forget about commitments and responsibilities or become preoccupied and distracted by other endeavors. Ask yourself: How would I feel if people were late to meet with me? Would I feel disregarded or disrespected?

Time

Notice what you do unconsciously or excessively throughout the day. Reclaim time that is poured into activities that don't add value to your life. Schedule your days to achieve balance. Incorporate healthy behaviors or outdoor exercise to counterbalance work. Make conscious choices about how you wish to spend your time.

Timelessness

Choose a time of day that works best for you and commit to a spiritual practice that allows for self-reflection and union with the divine. Perhaps select secular mindfulness practices to cultivate awareness of a universal quality such as compassion. Connect with nature in any way that feels right for you. Perform spontaneous acts of kindness and try to be of service to anyone in need.

12

Passion

Passion is commonly understood to be a strong, barely controllable emotion or a feeling of enthusiasm or excitement in regard to doing something specific, such as a creative endeavor. Although these general definitions are accurate, useful, and universal, those in recovery ought to consider another description for passion, as derived from its Latin root *pati*, which means "to suffer or endure pain."

In active addiction, suffering exists within the minds and hearts of those afflicted with dependent tendencies. Specific substances and behaviors are utilized to quell inner turmoil or angst, to alleviate pain—the alcoholic drinks; the addict ingests pills; the debtor gambles; the bulimic binges and purges; and so on. When addictive exploits are employed to remedy mental and emotional pain, anguish is exacerbated instead of eased, as any respite procured through dependence can only produce harmful, short-lived results and destabilize overall well-being.

Without healthy means to ascertain the causes and conditions for our suffering and wholesome options to transmute our pain, the effects of the trauma we are trying to address remain static or worsen. When attempts to avoid pain originate within cycles of agony perpetuated by unexamined thoughts and their consequent actions, lasting contentment is hardly possible. When we struggle to mitigate or eradicate suffering through detrimental activities, these efforts become ineffective and deplete our energy.

Six stages of active addiction illustrate how energy surges and dissipates and how emotions plateau and plummet before, during, and after engagement in self-defeating, habitual, destructive behaviors. Those who familiarize themselves with these ideas will comprehend the role passion plays in regard to recovery.

1. Preoccupation: We obsessively think about what we will do, when and how we will do it, and how we will get away with it. We are excited and anticipate what is to come.
2. Acquisition: We buy a bottle of alcohol, acquire certain substances, or plan and confirm dependent activities. We are anxious and no longer present. We are desirous of instant relief that seems imminent.
3. Anticipation: We experience a sense of euphoria just before the first drink, hit of a substance, or enactment of a behavior. We feel a lack of control. We are now unlikely to stop ourselves on our own power.
4. Acting out: We consume our drug of choice or realize our chosen activities. We feel relief. We feel out of control. We

become self-absorbed. Awareness of morality slips away from us.

5. Letdown: We experience a reduction of the effects from acting out as synthetic or natural chemicals leave our body. We feel emotional responses—sadness, depression, a lack of purpose. We feel physical consequences— imbalance, trembling, exhaustion, sweating, nausea.

6. Aftermath: We are emotionally exhausted, physically hungover, mentally depleted, and spiritually drained. We feel a need to clean up our messes or troubles or lie and cover up our behaviors. We feel guilt, remorse, shame, hopelessness, and perhaps suicidal. We feel enslaved to our addiction.

Imagine if the energy disbursed throughout these stages were instead harnessed and reallocated toward a higher purpose. Imagine if the thought processes that precede and sustain these stages were transmuted and the intellect could be utilized in a meaningful manner to some other end. Imagine if the intensity of suffering inherent in active addiction were substantiated in a new and wonderful life in recovery, within which passion no longer defines pain but purpose.

PRACTICING PASSION

According to Ayurvedic and yogic traditions, awareness of the *pancha mahabhutas*, or five great elements—earth, water, fire, air, space—is essential for optimum health and wholeness for all life-forms. When the interplay of these elements and their individual yet interdependent characteristics is harmonious, energy flows properly within the human body and balance is achieved throughout the cosmos.

Each element and its contribution to collective wellness is crucial for personal balance and interpersonal relations; however, *agni*, or fire, is responsible for transforming energy that has become inert or stuck. When energy is blocked, diminished, or misused at the physical or metaphysical level, awareness of agni transforms and redirects it from adaptation and healing. When energy is transmuted through cognizance of agni, health issues are rectified and *vikriti*, or various states of physical, physiological, and psychological illnesses—including addiction—can be prevented and treated.

Agni resides at the *manipura chakra*, or navel center. When metaphorical and genuine heat is created and sustained within the solar plexus region of the body, stagnant energy is converted into dynamic prana, or life-force energy, and redistributed throughout the body to achieve quantitative states of balance and health.

The following yogic practices optimize awareness of agni and stoke its proverbial and passionate fire within the belly. These suggestions also honor *svabhavoparamavada*, an Ayurvedic assertion that the body eliminates disease and heals itself when properly supported and balanced through regular and healthy breathing, exercise, meditation, and similar naturopathic protocols.

Kapalabhati, or Breath of Fire

Sit cross-legged on level ground, or sit upright in a chair. Rest your hands on your knees or in your lap. Lengthen your spine. Fix your gaze on a spot in front of you. Breathe all the air out of your lungs with an extended exhale. Seal your lips. Take an inhale through your nose. Exhale through your nostrils with short, successive, uninterrupted, repetitive bursts of air. With each exhale through your nose, draw your navel toward your spine. Continue this pattern for thirty seconds, then breathe regularly. Notice if your belly feels warm. Notice if you feel more energized or empowered.

Points of focus: Imagine how a dog might pant and find a similar rhythm as you send air out through the nostrils. The inhale will occur naturally as you find a pace that works for you. If you get fatigued or tired, slow down. If you get dizzy or lightheaded, stop and rest. If you wish to continue for more than thirty seconds, choose another time frame that feels appropriate.

Yogi Bicycle

Lie down on your back on a yoga mat or flat surface. Interlace your fingers behind your head. Bring your knees toward your chest. Extend your right leg and draw your right elbow toward your left knee. Return to a neutral position. Extend your left leg and draw your left elbow toward your right knee. Repeat these movements as you count to fifty, or choose a number of repetitions that best suits your practice.

Points of focus: Extend through your heel as each leg straightens. Spread your toes on both feet throughout the movements. Draw your navel down toward the spine as you lift one shoulder blade at a time off the mat. Find a steady pace that you can maintain. Don't pull at your head or neck, or force your elbows toward your knees. Allow your hands to act as a basket or nest to support your head and neck.

Trataka, **or Gazing Steadily**

Find a quiet space for meditation. Sit comfortably with your spine elongated. Light a candle and place it in front of you. Close your eyes. Take three deep, mindful breaths to anchor your awareness in the present moment. Open your eyes and gaze at the base of the flame. Focus on your in-breath and out-breath. Notice the interdependence of light, shadow, and darkness. After three minutes, close your eyes again. Locate the image of the flame within your mind. Harness the power of fire to incinerate fears and control issues that reside within your mind and body. Use the power of an inner flame to alchemize things in your life that stand in the way of recovery. Open your eyes when you are ready. Notice if your mind feels concentrated. Notice if your body feels strengthened. Safely extinguish the candle.

Points of focus: Darken the room or space where you will do this meditation. Use a natural, unscented candle. Maintain a safe distance between your body and the flame. If tears come, allow this process to cleanse and purify the eyes. If the eyes become uncomfortable, close them or use a tissue to gently absorb moisture.

Agni Mudra, **or Fire Seal**

Find a comfortable seat. Take five conscious breaths to bring your mind home to your body. Relax your shoulders. Relax your arms. Relax your hands. Make a fist with your right hand and extend the thumb upward. Open your left hand and place it in front of you with the palm open. Place your right hand inside your left. Cultivate stillness for five minutes as you hold and contemplate this gesture.

Points of focus: Recognize that a *mudra* is a gesture as an energetic lock or seal. Recognize that the right thumb represents the element of fire. Recognize that fire burns away impurities. Recognize that the power of fire resides within the body. Recognize that you have the power within you to change limiting beliefs and conditioned behaviors.

Japa, or Repetition Chanting

Find a comfortable, seated position. Familiarize yourself with the bija or seed sound *Ram*, which corresponds with the *manipura*, or navel chakra. Place one or both hands over your belly. Visualize energy swirling at this region beneath your hands. Soften your gaze or close your eyes. Relax your jaw. Begin to chant the syllable *Ram*. Find a recitation style and pace that feel natural to you. Relax your body and allow for organic movements if they arise. Chant *Ram* for three minutes or more, or use a yogic mala bead necklace and chant *Ram* as you touch each of the 108 beads. Stop chanting and find silence. Take three deep, belly breaths and feel the rise and fall of your abdomen beneath your hands. If your eyes are closed, open them. Internalize the affirmations: "I am strong," or "I am powerful," or "I can and will take risks to change my circumstances."

Points of focus: Recognize that the word *chakra* can be translated as "wheel of energy." Recognize that chanting moves energy throughout the body and redistributes it appropriately. Notice if your mind feels clearer as a result of this practice. Notice if your body feels energized and regulated.

LET'S MAKE THIS PERSONAL

Where does your energy go each day? What do you prioritize and spend time doing? How can you maximize the distribution of your personal energy? Where can you invest your energy and love to create collective healing or transformation?

What do you do for your mind and body to remain healthy? What practices help you to uplift your life and spirit? How do you find balance? How can you show others what you do to remain well so they can know and achieve wellness?

What are you passionate about? What are your deep, driving desires? What do you believe you are here to do with your life? What can you do each day to live your life with enthusiasm and determination? How can you share your passion with others?

Where in your life do you suffer? How much time do you spend in various manifestations of suffering, such as sorrow, unkindness, selfishness? How can you transform pain or misery into something useful or purposeful? How can you keep your recovery fresh, exciting, and joyful? How can the integrity of your recovery inspire others on their journey?

13

Presence

Recovery happens in the present moment. Healing and transformation happen in the present moment. Joy and happiness are experienced in the present moment. Sadness and anger are felt in the present moment. Life is lived in the present moment.

When we become intimate with the present moment, we experience a sense of groundedness. We feel a sense of home and belonging. We discover the truth of our circumstances. We understand what we can do to positively alter our thoughts and actions. We comprehend how to enrich our recovery and uplift the lives of others.

When we are unable to anchor our awareness in the present moment, regret or shame may overtake us if we contemplate the past, and fear or anxiety may dominate our thoughts if we ponder the future. When we live life through the lens of previous experiences, we recycle old feelings and can find ourselves unable to generate new emotions or enjoy original moments. When we live life through the lens of projection or in anticipation of what may come, mental congestion impedes our ability to identify solutions for our immediate concerns or challenges.

The only time we have to learn and grow is *now*. The only time we have to amend what needs to be amended is *now*. The only time we have to be useful to others is *now*. The only time we have to fulfill our destiny is *now*.

In recovery, we must address the nature of our relationship with the present moment if we are to know calm, balance, and peace. Examining how we nourish and protect the mind, body, and spirit in the present moment can lead us to hopefulness, resilience, and unity. We must look at how we think, speak, and act in the present moment if we are to realize that change is possible and our lives have meaning and purpose.

PRACTICING PRESENCE

The Yoga Sutras of Patanjali begin with the aphorism *Atha yoga anushasanam*, which can be translated as "Now, the teachings of yoga." The first word of this first sutra—*atha*, or "now"— signifies how essential present-moment awareness is if spiritual aspirants are to evolve along a yogic path. This use of the word *atha* is intentional and indispensable. It commands our attention. It leaves no room for misinterpretation as it elucidates the eternal truth that now is the only moment wherein we learn, grow, and transform our lives.

We can't practice yoga yesterday. We don't practice yoga tomorrow. Yesterday is gone, and tomorrow is not yet here. We practice yoga in the reality of now. We can't live life yesterday. We don't live life tomorrow. We live life in the reality of now. We can't get sober yesterday. We don't get sober tomorrow. We get sober in the reality of now.

Many people in active addiction engage in harmful behaviors to avoid the present moment. The reality of now is hardly a place people who suffer from shame and regret or depression and loneliness wish to reside. The present moment can be a painful place to be in for those who suffer from sorrow and anxiety or self-loathing and hopelessness. However, the present moment is where life happens and where all things exist. It is the only place where we can face the demons of dependence and discover the salvation of prajna, or deep insight, garnered through proper discernment.

Yes, grief resides in the present moment, but so does joy. Hatred lives in the present moment, but so does love. Sadness abides in the present moment, but so does happiness. If fear is in the present moment, so is faith. Death and rebirth coexist in the present moment. Addiction and recovery are both alive in the present moment.

Within the sanctity of the present moment we encounter things as they are, yet we often see things as we choose to see them. When we confront and name our emotions and resolve problematic issues in the present moment, freedom is possible. When we encounter and embrace unwholesome experiences and accept personal improvement in the present moment, inner peace is possible. When we meet inner circumstances and honor discomfort in the present moment, contentment is possible. When we stand our ground and make good use of trustworthy spiritual solutions in the present moment, happiness is possible. When we light a lamp of awareness to illuminate darkness in the present moment or untether ourselves from harmful situations and relationships in the present moment or act with courage amid doubt and distress in the present moment, recovery is alive and well in the present moment.

Whenever we utilize developmental and spiritual practices that support recovery in the reality of now, the mind holds on to its autonomy and our thoughts are imbued with intelligence and inspiration. Our words become intentional and clear and create healthy boundaries. Our actions originate from the vigor of a healthy body. Our spirit offers solace and solutions to those afflicted by the cruel and blinding forces of addiction. Below are suggestions to cultivate awareness of the present moment.

Past-Present-Future Meditation

Find a comfortable, seated position. Inhale and silently repeat "Inhale, present moment." Exhale and silently repeat "Exhale, present moment." Complete this cycle five times to pair awareness of the breath with the present moment. Next, inhale and silently repeat "Inhale, present moment." Exhale and silently repeat "Exhale, the past." Complete this cycle five times to establish present-moment awareness with each inhale and release attachment to the past with every exhale. Next, inhale and silently repeat "Inhale, present moment." Exhale and silently repeat "Exhale, the future." Complete this cycle five times to solidify present-moment awareness with each inhale and send away future concerns with every exhale. Next, inhale and silently repeat "Inhale, present moment." Exhale and silently repeat "Exhale, present moment." Complete this cycle five times to fortify the quality of your presence in the reality of now with each inhale and exhale.

Note: Once you are familiar with the instructions for this meditation, close your eyes as you practice. Personalize your inhales and exhales throughout this exercise to customize your relationship with the present moment. With inhales in the present moment, realize where you are and what you feel: "I am sitting outside" or "I am grateful." With exhales for the past, acknowledge what has already happened within your day: "I talked with a friend this morning" or "I am no longer at the office." With exhales for the future, realize what has not yet happened within your day: "I will eat dinner later" or "I will take a yoga class tonight."

Flower Contemplation

Choose a flower and find a relaxed posture. Hold the flower in your hands. Contemplate its colors, shape, and size. Feel its texture. Realize the flower is a miracle of nature. Realize that sunshine, rain, and soil have contributed to the manifestation of the flower. Realize the flower began as a seed. Realize the flower was a bud before it blossomed. Realize the flower will one day return to the earth. Raise the flower to your nose and inhale. Find gratitude for its fragrance. Place the flower aside or hold it within your hands. Close your eyes. Meditate on the essence of the flower. Visualize its colors, shape, and size. Internalize the qualities of the flower: resilience, beauty, uniqueness. Internalize how you share these qualities with the flower. Reflect on the life span of the flower and the nature of impermanence. Reflect on your life span and the nature of your impermanence. Reflect on the significance of appreciating all things as they are in the present moment. Remain in contemplation for five minutes or more. Open your eyes and return to the reality of now.

Tadasana, or Mountain Pose

Stand with your feet hip-distance apart. Root down through all four corners of your feet—the mound under the big toe, the mound under the small toe, the inner heel, the outer heel. Draw earth energy up through the souls of your feet. Feel this energy rise up through your ankles, shins, and knees. Feel this energy climb up through your thighs and hips. Feel this energy travel into your belly and heart. Bring your hands together in prayer position at your heart to harness this energy. Relax your shoulders. Broaden the space across your collarbones. Lift your heart to the sky. Bring your chin parallel to the earth. Draw your navel toward your spine to activate your core. Tuck your tailbone toward your heels. Lift your kneecaps and engage your thighs. Choose a focal point or close your eyes. Take ten deep breaths in this posture. Feel a sense of groundedness. Feel the qualities of solidity, strength, and presence.

Inhabiting the Present Moment

When we are not present or at home in the reality of now, the windows of the mind are left ajar and doorways into the body remain open. When we are not present, addiction and its minions—bewilderment and melancholy, paranoia and perversity, lethargy and despondency—creep into our thought forms, enter our bodies, and sever our contact with the spirit. When we are not present, disease infiltrates all layers of the self— mental, emotional, physical, and spiritual.

Addiction is an exceptional thief. It knows whom to attack, how its victims are weak, where they are vulnerable, and when to steal their valuables. Addiction is watchful and only enters vacant mental spaces, seeks neglected bodies hitched to distracted minds, and pursues souls that are unaware of their divine dimension.

When addiction sneaks into our lives, it oversees the management of our interiority and systematically destroys our well-being. It distorts our perception, which ruins personal relationships. It appropriates our time, which affects peace of mind. It skews our sense of personal safety, which prohibits awareness of purpose. It snuffs out our inner light, which diminishes our outer life.

Addiction can't penetrate the sanctuary of self when we are at home in the reality of now to defend ourselves from invasion. It can't overwhelm the unified mind, body, and spirit in the present moment. It can't conquer a person who is inhabited by peace, purpose, and presence.

When we remain rooted in the present moment, our composure bears witness to the qualities of steadfastness and discipline. Our prayers promote individual and interactive harmony. Our meditations supply revelations and solutions to all troubles and vexations. Our presence brings blessings of benevolence, impartiality, and encouragement to those in and out of recovery.

We may miss our entire lives if we can't comprehend the significance of presence. We may become bystanders to things we are meant to see, hear, and feel if we can't develop the ability to accept things as they are within the reality of now. We may never say what needs to be said or do what needs to be done if we can't humbly and completely embrace the present moment.

LET'S MAKE THIS PERSONAL

Are you comfortable in the present moment? Do you seek outer distractions or engage in specific behaviors to avoid the present moment?

In which areas of your life can you be more present for yourself? How can you honor the gift of life as it is right now? How can you be grateful for all you have right now?

Within personal relationships, how can you be more attentive to others? More selfless with your time? More understanding? More loving and compassionate?

How can you honor your mind, body, and spirit within the reality of now? How can you observe the simplicity and magnanimity of nature within the reality of now? How can you incorporate moments of stillness and silence into your recovery within the reality of now?

What can you do today to improve your means of concentration and communication? What can you say today that needs to be said? What can you do today that needs to be done?

Can you recognize all the wonders of life available in the present moment? Can you feel moments of grace within the present moment? Can you seize opportunities to love and serve others in the present moment?

Can you believe that your fate can only be claimed in the present moment? Personal brokenness can only be healed in the present moment? Collective rejuvenation can only happen in the present moment? Transformation stories can only be written in the present moment? God or any higher power of individual understanding can only demonstrate omnipotence in the present moment?

14

Willingness

Within recovery, willingness is the readiness to do something constructive at any time to ensure the security of our mental, emotional, physical, and spiritual health. It means making ourselves perpetually available in ways that are functional, helpful, and positive. It is an enduring capacity to do what needs to be done to bring estimable acts to fruition.

Recovery is a matter of life and death for people who have suffered the misfortunes of active addiction. Mistakes in recovery are costly, and wrong actions can be fatal. We can't take chances with short-lived moments of readiness, minimal preparation, or lackluster enthusiasm. We can't allow personal biases or obstinacy to impede our development. We must be determined to do whatever it takes to achieve physical and emotional sobriety, mental coherency, and spiritual awareness.

Willingness is a neutral principle; it is applicable and advantageous within both positive and negative situations. If an active alcoholic desperately needs to drink, willingness fuels their thoughts and actions so they succeed in their undertakings regardless of consequences. For example, they will go crosstown in the middle of the night for a drink, steal money to pay for alcohol, and lie about their whereabouts. If a sober alcoholic desperately needs to remain sober, willingness will propel them toward recovery, no matter the circumstances. For example, they will attend a twelve-step meeting, contact sober friends for advice or suggestions, and make good use of prayer, meditation, and other spiritual tools.

When we can recognize willingness as unbiased, we can see how it eliminates negative habits and benefits all aspects of recovery. However, we must first know what we wish to achieve within our lives before we can profit from willingness. If we do not know what we desire or why we may be moving in a certain direction, we can't in good conscience proceed toward an unknown destination and hope for a satisfactory outcome.

When we establish personal goals for what we plan to do with sobriety, willingness sustains our efforts to remain sober. When we nourish ourselves with the power of volition, willingness infuses our thoughts with ingenuity and our actions with valor. When we aspire to transform our lives and the lives of others, willingness influences the efficacy of our recovery and substantiates our existence.

INTENTIONALITY AND WILLINGNESS

Within yogic philosophy, the term *sankalpa* can be interpreted as "intention." It is a direction or goal for our practice and life. It is something we hope to achieve. It is a feeling or quality we can cultivate and set within ourselves. It is something we can return to and focus on when the mind wanders or becomes restless. It is also something beneficial or devotional that we can offer to others.

When we look at the etymology of the Sanskrit word *sankalpa*, *san* can be defined as "highest truth" and *kalpa* can be interpreted as "vow or rule to follow." Sankalpa can ultimately be viewed as a call to awakening when we commit to know who we truly are and uncompromisingly strive to accomplish what we are here to do with our lives.

Imagine a traveler is headed toward a distant or unfamiliar location. Without a map or means to navigate such a journey, the destination may be difficult to reach. By land, automobile drivers enter addresses into a global positioning system (GPS) device. By air, pilots use radar and advanced instruments to safely fly planes. By sea, captains command boats with chronometers, charts, and other reliable methods.

Sankalpa is an inner atlas that guides people toward a predetermined destination in life. Without an idea of where we wish to go and what we hope to accomplish, we may veer off course, mismanage our time, and lose our bearings. We may hesitate to advance when obstacles appear in our path. We may abandon our voyage when coordinates and objectives are unclear or conditions seem insurmountable.

When we honor a sankalpa, an internal itinerary prompts us to utilize proficiencies, actualize desires, and fulfill our svadharma, or personal purpose. When we set aside *alasya*, or laziness, and adopt *iccha*, or willingness, as a consistent way of being, inherent blueprints outline a plan for living that corresponds with our *prakriti*, or individual constitution. When we realize the body is our vehicle within this lifetime and the heart is our compass, willingness becomes the source of energy that allows us to encounter and overcome each twist and turn of our human journey.

DISCOVERING INTENTIONS AND DEVELOPING WILLINGNESS

Within the yogic tradition, there is a threefold practice that can help us discover sankalpa—*sravana*, or listening; *manana*, or reflection; and *nididhyasana*, or meditation. When these three interdependent methods for self-discovery are observed conscientiously, *avidya*, or ignorance, is dispelled, and inner wisdom is revealed in its absence. Additionally, willingness to realize positive personal ambitions develops in the lives of those whose efforts are diligent and sincere.

Sravana suggests listening to teachings that lead us toward knowledge of our divine nature, awareness of our oneness with all things, and knowingness of our unique place within the universe.

Here are some ways to practice this: Attend classes, lectures, or workshops with teachers who guide students toward their inmost nature. Read religious, spiritual, or inspirational literature. Listen to recordings that elucidate the inner workings of the mind. Become willing to hear stirrings within the heart and promptings from an internal teacher.

. . .

Manana suggests internalizing what is gleaned from spiritual instruction and trustworthy teachers or mentors. It is to explore the dimensions of *vichara*, or self-inquiry, and *svadhyaya*, or self-study. It is to contemplate the individualization of relative truth in accordance with the omnipresence of absolute truth.

Here are some ways to practice this: Utilize silence, stillness, and solitude to reflect on what you hear and absorb through sravana. Discern the usefulness of universal or spiritual knowledge. Discover what is true within your heart. Become willing to allow heartfelt wisdom to emanate from the center of your being.

Nididhyasana suggests meditation as a method to fully integrate self-realizations attained through sravana and manana. As a result, conviction of inner truth becomes solidified and manifests as concentrated thought, compassionate or loving speech, and right action.

Here are some ways to practice this: Meditate on what you absorb through sravana and what you understand through manana. Visualize how you will act on these insights. Become willing to naturally and fully realize your visions.

WILLINGNESS TO SAFEGUARD RECOVERY

Addiction is willing to hurt anyone and anything. It is willing to humiliate and torture its victims. It is willing to make use of psychological and physical warfare and force itself into the minds and bodies of those who can't adequately or properly defend themselves. It is willing to inflict pain on any sufferer, anywhere in the world, within any moment of any day.

The intention of addiction is to seek and destroy. It knows its reasons for being. It is not confused about why it is here or what it wishes to accomplish. It does not waver from its aims or hesitate to demolish anything that stands in its path. It stops at nothing to propagate myriad forms of misery in the lives of its victims.

If we are unwilling to become intentional within our lives, we may not fare well against the unrelenting assaults of addiction. If we are unwilling to identify and pursue our vocations, we may remain disoriented or directionless and fail to rise above the pains and procedures of habitual dependence. If we are unwilling to avoid emotional stagnancy, mental laxity, and spiritual stasis, we may not synchronize inner cognizance with outer direction to achieve continuous sobriety and lasting recovery.

LET'S MAKE THIS PERSONAL

Do you know where you are going with your life? Do you have clarity about your purpose? Do you know who you are here to be?

Are you willing to listen to inner and outer wisdom? To internalize universal principles or spiritual teachings? To meditate on things that can change your life and the lives of others?

Are you willing to practice fidelity in regard to recovery? To remain single-minded and untiringly dedicated to the unfolding of recovery? To help others along their path to recovery?

Are you willing to examine or dispel judgments and opinions you may have about addiction, recovery, or spirituality? Are you willing to adopt new beliefs or have new experiences with life?

Are you willing to identify causes and conditions that underlie your tendencies to drink, use drugs, or partake in harmful behaviors?

Are you willing to subdue agitations within the mind, heal past traumas, and neutralize personal triggers?

Are you willing to seek assistance, consider helpful suggestions, and learn from your mistakes?

Are you willing to develop indwelling predispositions, intuitive capabilities, and unique strengths?

Are you willing to share what you learn within your recovery and life with others in need of guidance or camaraderie?

What can you do today to identify your intentions and nurture your aspirations? To align inner cognizance with outer surroundings? To express the life you are here to live?

15

Humility

Humility in recovery means recognizing that we have reached the extent of our own power. It is affirming that our capability to overcome addiction and its various factions is limited; our ability to heal ourselves and others is limited; and our capacity to self-transform and bear witness to the miracles of recovery is limited.

Humility is a retiring of personal intelligence, willful effort, and human resources in favor of unknown entities and immutable, spiritual realities. It is to dismantle self-constructed mental scaffoldings that uphold edifices of individuality. It is abandoning emotional propensities that preserve illusions of uniqueness. It means to bow with reverence before seemingly unsolvable dilemmas and renounce personal authority to providential or cosmic counsel.

When humility becomes part of recovery, we are freed from the complexes of superiority, inferiority, and equality and no longer oscillate between states of self-importance, desperation, or complacency. We trust that right actions indeed cause right effects, and we no longer claim ownership of our achievements or misfortunes, evaluate our successes and failures, or tally the wins and losses of others. We accept praise and criticism evenly, resign from the roles of victor and victim, and react corresponding to the unpredictability and impermanent nature of people, places, and things.

When pride, vanity, and similar impediments to humility no longer exacerbate our addictions with temporal, mental responses and hasty or futile physical reactions, inner doubts and outer criticisms evaporate, and divides between depression and happiness, agitation and calm, and dependency and recovery can be negotiated. When selfishness and self-glorification are yielded and replaced with prudence and reticence, our disposition is rightly tempered, and we respond proportionately to positive, negative, and neutral circumstances. When egocentric expectations and desired outcomes are fully renounced, self-effacement clarifies all aspects of the mind and a doorway opens to the inner sanctum of the heart, where the riches of recovery await discovery.

THE HEART AND HUMILITY

Within yogic philosophy, the term *hridaya* represents the spiritual heart. Hridaya is the inner shrine within the depths of the human heart where our mystical essence or divine nature resides. It is the home of cosmic consciousness, the place where Creator and creation are unified, the ineffable abode of universal love and infinite truth. It is the secret *guha*, or cave, within the heart where humble yet magnanimous abilities to think, see, listen, speak, and act with compassion are sourced from a vast reservoir of ultimate wisdom.

When we familiarize ourselves with the natural purity of hridaya, all vestiges of self are attenuated and removed from our character. We no longer suffer oppression from conditions that agitate the mortal mind, nor are we distraught in situations that unsettle the subjectivity of human emotionality. We no longer entertain or act upon desires or dependences that originate from our physiological, earthly disposition, and we become impartial and equanimous when enticements or perturbations are encountered.

Hridaya is the innermost place within all beings where nothingness and godliness are experienced simultaneously. It is where we carry the reminiscences and energies of past and present beloveds, teachers, and friends. It is where all humankind are viewed as kin, and all living things are regarded as fellow sojourners on an internal and eternal, individual yet collective path toward becoming *jivanmuktas*, or liberated living beings.

If we wish to be emancipated from the bondage of addiction, we must acquaint ourselves with the conceptual and qualitative states of hridaya and allow our senses to be respectively attuned. We must personalize the intrinsic value of hridaya so our undertakings become a perfect balance of offering and receiving. We must allow our conception of hridaya to become embodied so our thoughts and actions become synonymous and beneficial, and covetousness, attachment, and conceit can be forever removed from our consciousness.

LET'S MAKE THIS PERSONAL

The following sets of questions guide practitioners toward an awareness of hridaya and comprehensively acclimate our faculties for greater humility and compassion toward ourselves and others. These questions are self-reflective by nature so that we can identify how we are vulnerable, insecure, and self-conscious in order to be able to recognize these and similar qualities in others. When we detect and name our weaknesses and imperfections, empathy, kindness, and additional altruistic tendencies will arise within us as we encounter unwholesomeness, brokenness, and boastfulness in others. When we viscerally and palpably know personal sufferings and humiliations, we will acknowledge and revere the centermost place in others where these things are perfected through the primacy of unity.

Think from the Heart

Can you contemplate how your addictions or personal hardships provide opportunities to know humility and spiritual growth? Can you disengage from the misery of past sufferings and release attachment to future concerns or worries? Can you acknowledge your shortcomings and the misgivings of others as manifestations of inner anguish? Can you honor sorrow and pain as teachers? Can you imagine being totally emancipated from the bondage of self? Can you recall the names and faces of friends who have helped you find happiness and freedom and send them thoughts of gratitude? Can you consider all beings as imperfect yet worthy of love and understanding? Can you consider that all beings have a specific purpose, unique talents, and a poignant place within the order of the universe? Can you think of ways to encourage the actualization of inherent, positive potentiality within yourself and others?

See from the Heart

How do you see yourself when you look into a mirror? Are you complimentary or critical? Can you look beyond the physical body to see the truth of your existence? Can you see into your spiritual heart? Can you see your vital role in the continual unfoldment of nature? Can you see that you are a child of the cosmos and your presence sustains the ritam, or cosmic rhythm, of life? Can you see that others are also children of the cosmos? Can you view addictions and similar afflictions as opportunities for all living things to individually learn and grow and collectively heal and transform? Can you recognize your joys and the joys of others? Can you behold your pain and the pain of others? Can you envision your life without disagreeable dependences or destructive habits? Can you visualize being a friend or helper to anyone who lacks companionship or support? Can you picture your present and future relationships as healthy and beneficial to all persons involved? Can you look into the mirror of life and see freedom for anyone who suffers from addiction, narcissism, and similar conditions that impede the maturation of humility?

Listen from the Heart

Can you hear intuitive or divine thoughts and understand these messages? Can you hear past or present cries of suffering from within your mind and body and answer these calls for help? Can you listen to stillness within your soul? Can you discern noble silence in prayer and meditation? Can you determine when your inner or outer speech betrays your emotions and feelings? Can you recognize that truthfulness has an unmistakable resonance? Can you recognize that dishonesty has a distinctive timbre? Can you listen to and appreciate the intonation of your inhale and exhale as they nourish your body? Can you recognize moments of silence between your breaths? Can you detect a tone or quality within the voice or breaths of others? Can you hear when others may be asking for help, love, or compassion when they audibly sigh, uncomfortably laugh, or silently cry? Can you listen to others with peaceful objectivity so they can unburden what weighs heavy on their minds and hearts? Can you be a citadel of compassion amid silent or noisy moments with others? Can you hear the cries of the world and take action to alleviate these pains?

Speak from the Heart

How would you define your personal, human qualities? How would you begin to express the totality of your spiritual essence? When you speak about yourself, are your words truthful and supportive? Which mantras or affirmations pervade your mentality? Are you honest when you convey your feelings and emotions? Is your speech congruent with your reality? How do you inwardly or outwardly speak about others? What is the quality of your tone when you address others? Can your speech remedy the ills of others within your home or community? Can you recognize that your words have the power to heal or harm? Can you vow to be mindful when you internally or externally speak? Can you express wisdom from your heart within personal conversations and all interactions? Can you utilize sacred silence for heart-centered communication? Can your words—inaudible or audible—be filled with reverence, praise, and modesty today?

THE VALUE OF A HUMBLE HEART

When we become aware of the unparalleled properties of the heart, harmony and wholeness result, and addiction is unable to separate our mind from our body and spirit, divide our human cognition from divine perception, or disconnect any being from the safety and security of fellowship with other beings.

When we seek refuge within the sacred stronghold of hridaya and endeavor to understand its immeasurable qualities, humility protects us from all external nemeses and internal neuroses. Self-contempt and perplexity are forsaken. Selfish desires and vanity are eliminated from our temperament. Meekness replaces self-condemnation. Defenselessness clarifies our perspective. Feelings of inner or outer discontent become transitory. Personal objectives are no longer spiteful or wretched. Loneliness can't penetrate our inner life. Hindrances signify opportunities for growth. Boasting and complaining are abandoned. Spiritual inquisitiveness directs our daily considerations. Self-abnegation outlines our path to freedom. Despair and unknowingness no longer afflict our conscious or unconscious thoughts.

When we earnestly consider how the heart and humility nourish our thoughts, words, actions, and senses, continuous recovery naturally manifests as we abstain from harming the vessel by which the heart travels and no longer poison the mind, desecrate the body, or dishonor the spirit. When we comprehend the mutually beneficial relationship between the heart and re-covery, we commit to its preservation and abide by the perpetuity of its evolution. When we share our hearts and recovery with those who seek healing and transformation, our aspirations are empathetic, our energy is unpretentious, and our knowledge is trustworthy.

16

Humanity

The concept of humanity is indispensable in addiction recovery if we are to develop and maintain personal recovery. Humanity can be viewed as awareness of oneness with others on similar paths to recovery, healing, and transformation. It means to regard all such persons as fellow travelers without bias about their backgrounds and habits or judgments about their methods and practices. It is to overlook outer differences so that we can connect at the subtle, human level of feeling or emotion, through cognizance of shared ways of thinking, speaking, and acting.

When well-meaning clients in addiction treatment centers first meet one another, they typically ask, "What was your drug of choice?" or "What did you do to end up here?" If answers to these queries and subsequent questions and conversations do not transcend surface-level curiosity to include exploratory inquiries and disclosures of personal truths, clients remain estranged and recovery becomes difficult to sustain. On the flip side, when we honestly and humbly identify as human beings who may suffer from alcoholism, drug addiction, and other human vices and behaviors, rather than regard and label ourselves alcoholics, addicts, or similar designations, a humane and societal need for love and understanding becomes apparent and can be offered and received accordingly.

When personal, human challenges and difficulties are properly viewed as communal characteristics of our humanness rather than preferential quirks or premeditated, individualized attempts to promulgate harm or sorrow, we find ourselves in a united struggle with those in similar predicaments. When we can recognize human idiosyncrasies as evolutionary and ubiquitous, rather than random and subjectively calculated, our recovery materializes through this coherent and straightforward method of humanization. When we individually and collectively accept our situations and take right actions toward changing behaviors that can be injurious, spiritual development becomes possible and all humankind benefits within present civilizations and future generations.

When humanity is considered a tool for harmonization within a program of recovery, we discover why we think what we think within the human mind, feel what we feel within the human body, and experience what we experience within the human life. We also learn to value what others in active addiction or recovery may think within their human minds, feel what they feel within their human bodies, and experience what they experience within their human lives. Through these cognitive processes of personal and interpersonal investigation, patterns of thought, feeling, and experience emerge as common denominators within the lives of human beings who suffer from addiction. Through unity with other human beings who have analogous root causes and conditions that lead to negative or unhealthy behavior, solutions to transmute the stimuli lurking beneath addictions are discovered. And through reliance on the interdependent nature of humanity, pathways to healing and recovery are revealed when human minds, hearts, and souls are venerated as complementary, integrated, and inseparable.

YOGIC SPIRITUALITY AND HUMANITY

Namaste is a Sanskrit expression that has transcended traditional yogic cosmology and entered the modern lexicon of global language. Many people recognize this three-syllable word as a spiritual salutation and gesture, typically enacted by uttering the word while placing the hands together in *anjali mudra*, or prayer position, at the heart. In regard to humanity and recovery, let's examine the etymological relevance of the word *namaste* to learn how this ancient term synchronizes divine and human perspectives to elevate contemporary ways of thinking, communicating, and acting. Let's also assess the potential of its harmonizing effects on mental, emotional, and physical aspects of recovery.

Nama denotes all of the following: to bow; to bend or stoop; to yield or submit; to give away. *As* represents "I" or "me." *Te* signifies "you" or "other." Thus, a translation of *namaste* could be "I bow to you," which implies eradication of the individual self as unification with the other occurs through an act of surrender. To further support this interpretation, if the word *nama* is dissected, we learn that *na* indicates "negation" and *ma* symbolizes "mine." When these two sounds are conjoined, the connotation is complete cessation of egoism as the entirety of our divine and human selves can be perceived within the divine and human reflection of others.

At the end of a yoga class, a teacher and students characteristically bow their heads and join their palms together at the heart while repeating "namaste." If asked what this word or ritual represents, instructors often offer a derivative of the statement: "The Divine Light in me honors the Divine Light in you." This explanation suffices to help practitioners begin to feel the spiritual import of namaste. However, if the humanistic connotations of namaste are not equally explored, the heart may not fully open to honor the inseparable duality of spirituality and humanity.

Within yogic philosophy, the human body is viewed as the vessel by which the spirit travels within a lifetime. Without humanity, the Light—or Love, or God, or Highest Self, or any name attributed to the spark of divinity within all human beings—has no means to manifest upon the mortal plane of existence. If we fail to comprehend the value of humanity or discount its mental, emotional, and physical attributes, we can't expect to alchemize what is in need of transformation such as harmful personal patterns of thought, universal feelings and emotions that lead to addictive behavior, or irrational actions that create wreckage within the reality of now and in the future.

PRACTICING NAMASTE

To make use of the human imagination and divine intuition to personalize the benefits of namaste, find a comfortable seat and place your hands together at your heart. Set your thumbs lightly against your chest. Know that the mudra or gesture you have created with your hands is an energetic lock or seal. Know that when the mudra for namaste is created at the heart, our capacity to know and generate love, compassion, understanding, forgiveness, and similar positive traits is deepened.

Take five conscious breaths. Allow your mind to unite with your body and spirit. Bring awareness to your hands. Feel all fingers of your left hand merge with all fingers of your right hand. Contemplate that the number ten, according to numerology, signifies completion or perfection. Ponder that there are ten moral codes and self-disciplines outlined by Patanjali in the Yoga Sutras. You may also wish to recognize there are Ten Commandments in the Bible or that some Buddhist traditions recognize ten *paramitas*, or perfections.

Contemplate that the left side of the body represents femininity and the right side of the body represents masculinity. Intuit the marriage of these dualities at your heart. Recognize there is no longer a division between left or right, feminine or masculine. Recognize there is no longer discord between other polarities such as sun and moon, action and knowledge, theory and practice, inwardness or outwardness. Allow your heart to bear witness to these alliances. Feel the true meaning of the word *yoga*, which is "union."

Draw your chin toward your chest and slightly bow your head. Pause to cultivate inner silence and outer stillness. When you are ready, reflect on the personal intimacy and interpersonal immediacy of the following scenarios. Contemplate the intersection of humanity and spirituality within these situations. Recognize the prevalence of similarity within the actions and words of these exchanges.

Imagine a friend sits before you with their hands in prayer as they candidly pronounce: "The sadness and depression within me recognizes and embraces the sadness and depression in you."

What thoughts arise for you when you read or hear this statement? Can you feel validation in regard to the inner workings of your mind? Can you feel that another person understands the magnitude of your personal thoughts? Can you feel camaraderie as you process the details of your darkness or addiction?

Imagine another friend were to sit in front of you with their hands over their heart as they earnestly declare: "The fear in me sees and honors the fear in you."

What emotions arise within you as you read or hear this declaration? Can you feel as if a component of your mentality has been corroborated? Can you feel empathetically connected to someone or something other than yourself? Can you believe that fear could dissipate within the mind and heart as a result of this interaction?

Imagine a teacher or mentor bows their head in your direction as they fold their hands together in front of their heart and sympathetically share: "The anger and loneliness in me forgives the anger and loneliness in you."

What is your reaction as you read and hear this disclosure? Can you feel as if burdens and grievances could be released from your psyche? Can you feel as if certain places within your body where tension accumulates could be healed or restored? Can you believe that mental, emotional, and physical harmony is the birthright of all human beings?

Pause to consider additional thoughts, emotions, and sensations that you may feel as a result of this practice. Contemplate the universality of your interiority. Consider how you may offer solace to others through the embodiment of your experience.

17

Congruency

Congruency is the quality of being in alignment or in harmony with other things. It is a relative term and can't exist on its own. Just as mindfulness can't exist without a subject, such as mindfulness of breath; concentration can't exist without an object, such as concentration on a *drishti*, or focal point; and insight can't exist without an observation, such as insight about the nature of impermanence, congruency can't exist without associated concepts.

Inherent to the principle of congruency is relational dependence among conceptions, opinions, feelings, behaviors, and other things. When compatibility is established among positive categorizations and resultant routines are followed, order and balance likely result. When negative patterns are developed between any types of pairings and detrimental habits are established, conflict and chaos ensue. Therefore, congruency either helps or hinders recovery to the degree we focus on beneficial or disadvantageous things and the measure of our dedication throughout these processes.

To make good use of congruency, we must first analyze how certain conceptual combinations contribute to our mental, emotional, physical, and spiritual health. Next, we skillfully choose where to place our attention and consciously exert our energies so that we can receive personal and interpersonal benefits. Last, we become intentional when we commit to the preservation of individual practices and remain diligent as we engender a virtuous life in recovery and beyond.

Let's look at three fundamental pairings—thought-speech-action, mind-body-spirit, past-present-future—to explore the example of both positive and negative congruency in relation to recovery and how our views about these three paradigms influence overall well-being.

THOUGHT-SPEECH-ACTION

When positive thoughts are congruent with affirmative words and deeds, recovery unfolds organically and favorably. For example, imagine a sober man feels that he may take a drink and relapse. If he can pause to think about calling a mentor or trusted friend, make the call to talk about his feelings, and perhaps attend a twelve-step meeting or similar gathering to find supplemental support, he will likely maintain his sobriety. Contrarily, if the same man does not acknowledge his desire to drink and fails to communicate his feelings, he may act to satisfy rather than arrest his cravings, as negative thoughts produce congruent speech and action.

MIND-BODY-SPIRIT

When matters of the mind, body, and spirit are harmonious, recovery becomes synergistically ordered. For example, imagine a woman in recovery recognizes that her mind is racing beyond her control. If she can pause and choose to participate in a practice that unifies mind, body, and spirit—such as yoga—this solution will likely quiet her mind, relax and strengthen her body, and help her establish conscious contact with her spirit. On the other hand, if she disregards her experience of mental instability and does not remedy the situation, psychosomatic and physiological effects may include anxiety, shortness of breath, elevated heart rate, increased blood pressure, and an inability to achieve a higher state of consciousness or spiritual awareness.

PAST-PRESENT-FUTURE

When past, present, and future are viewed as a continuum of inextricably related moments, recovery is stabilized through conscientious accountability and experiential symmetry. For example, imagine a person in recovery suffers from depression and they desire to take illicit drugs to alleviate their symptoms. If they can pause and choose to analyze past traumas or similar root causes that may have contributed to the onset of their condition, they can glean insight into the nature of their malady, which will enable them to heal their past, manage their circumstances in the reality of now, and safeguard their recovery for the future. Contrarily, if they deny or regret past situations or disregard previously experienced emotions or feelings, they will be unlikely to find peace in the present moment or within the foreseeable future.

A YOGIC VIEW OF CONGRUENCY

From a yogic perspective, an examination of the Sanskrit term *vinyasa* can deepen our understanding of how congruency codifies and harmonizes all aspects of recovery. The prefix *vi-* can be defined as "special or sacred way." The suffix *-nyasa* means "to place or arrange." When these two words are conjoined to create the compound *vinyasa*, the essential need to place and arrange not only *asanas*, or poses, but all matters of life in a meaningful and congruous manner becomes evident.

Vinyasa as a style of yoga is characterized by intelligent and progressive sequencing that systematically and gradually guides students from one pose to the next through the synchronization of mindful movement and conscious breath. Every movement within a vinyasa practice is unique and transient as each phase or pose informs the next phase or series of postures. Every breath taken during a vinyasa practice sustains practitioners as the multidimensionality of existence is examined amid the regulation of inhalations for expansive actions and exhalations for contractive movements. And every moment of vinyasa practice is an opportunity to find balance between effort and stillness while inwardly and outwardly exploring the five yamas, or moral codes—nonharming, truthfulness, nonstealing, right use of energy, nongreed—and the five niyamas, or self-disciplines—purity, contentment, discipline, self-study, surrender to a higher power.

Vinyasa as a physical discipline is accessible to many practitioners since poses can be modified as needed and breath can be regulated as required. This style of bodily practice affords students ample opportunities to recognize how all physiological aspects of practice must correspond if negative circumstances such as injury and fatigue are to be avoided and positive rewards such as healing and vitality are to be received. However, if the ontological significance of vinyasa is not equally explored off the mat in the world, practitioners will hardly comprehend the fundamental and pragmatic essence of vinyasa in relation to congruency or receive the entirety of its benefits.

PRACTICING CONGRUENCY

Within tantric yoga traditions, *nyasa* describes practices whereby mental consciousness is rotated throughout the physical body and mantras, symbolic imagery, and spiritual concepts are placed at various energetic vortices and other locations. When attention is sequentially brought to different parts of the body in this manner, subtle layers of mind and body are awakened, and blockages and similar incongruences are cleared. As a result, *nadis*, or inner pathways, are opened and *shakti*—a divine, creative, harmonizing force of energy—can flow unobstructed and unify all levels of our being.

A popular form of nyasa is *yoga nidra*, or "yogic sleep." Within this restorative practice, students are guided toward a state of consciousness between waking and sleeping wherein healing, relaxation, and transformation are generated through the utilization of three disciplines: *pratyahara*, or sensory withdrawal, which eliminates external distractions; *pranayama*, or breath regulation, which quiets the mind; and *dharana*, or concentration, which develops single-pointed focus.

Below is a yoga nidra practice for congruency. You will mentally scan your body and place awareness at specific areas to unify thoughts, words, and actions. You will explore the virtue of gratitude to harmonize your mind, body, and spirit. And you will observe mindfulness techniques to recognize the causal nexus of past, present, and future.

Find a comfortable position, lying down on a mat or sitting in a chair. Find stillness. Inhale and feel where you are in the present moment; exhale and anchor your awareness in the reality of now. Take two more breaths in this manner. Allow your mind to settle. Allow your physical body to settle. Allow your innermost self or spirit to settle.

Think of what you would like to achieve during this exercise. Hold that thought or quality as a sankalpa, or intention, within your heart throughout the practice. You can also choose an affirmation, such as "All aspects of my being are congruent," and place this sentence or a similar belief at one or various locations throughout the body. After you choose an intention and/or affirmation, take a deep inhale; then exhale to continue the practice.

Bring awareness to your feet. Think of all the things your feet allow you to do: walk, run, hike, and more. Wiggle your toes. Circle your ankles. Send gratitude to your feet for places they have taken you in the past and places they will take you in the future. Thank your feet for holding you up and supporting you.

With awareness and gratitude at your feet, take an inhale; exhale, and release awareness from your feet.

Bring awareness to your legs. Think of all the things your legs allow you to do: practice yoga, ride a bicycle, dance, play sports, and more. Bring awareness to your shins, knees, thighs; calves, hamstrings. Send gratitude to your legs for their ability to maintain balance so that you do not fall. Thank your legs for their symmetry. Thank your ligaments, muscles, and bones for their coherence. With awareness and gratitude at your legs, take an inhale; exhale, and release awareness from your legs.

Bring awareness to your hands. Think of all the things your hands allow you to do: write, eat, cook, clean, care for children, pet animals, and more. Wiggle your fingers. Circle your wrists. Send thankfulness into your hands for all the work they do on your behalf. Thank your hands for each flower they have picked; each handshake they have shared; each mudra they have enacted. Thank your palms for their example of openness and peacefulness. With awareness and gratitude at your hands, take an inhale; exhale, and release awareness from your hands.

Bring awareness to your arms. Think of all the things your arms allow you to do: hug family members and dear friends; swim, climb trees, and more. What are some things your arms have helped you achieve? Can you send gratitude to your arms right now? Can you be grateful for your elbows? Biceps? Triceps? Shoulders? Can you remember the last thing you embraced fully with your arms? What will be the next thing you embrace within your open arms? With awareness and gratitude for your arms, take an inhale; exhale, and release awareness from your arms.

Bring awareness to your torso. Think of your stomach, gallbladder, intestines, liver, spleen, pancreas, kidneys, bladder, lungs, heart. Within your body, your organs keep you healthy and alive. Express gratitude: "Thank you, my heart, my lungs, my bladder, my kidneys, my pancreas, my spleen, my liver, my intestines, my gallbladder, my stomach. Thank you for sustaining my existence. Thank you for doing what you were created to do. Thank you for doing your job so well. Thank you for contributing to the miracle of my life." With awareness and gratitude at your torso and upon your internal organs, take an inhale; exhale, and release awareness from this area.

Bring awareness to your eyes. Think of all the shapes and colors that you get to see. Think about the last person you saw. Imagine the smiles of children, flowers in a garden, a sunrise or sunset. Send gratitude to your eyes for their ability to correctly and clearly portray the many wonders of life.

Bring awareness to your ears. Think of all the sounds that you get to hear. Think about friends laughing, ocean waves crashing, music playing. Send gratitude to your ears for allowing you to hear the sounds of all sentient beings and other beautiful things.

Bring awareness to your mouth. Think of all the ways your mouth helps you fully experience the world. Think about foods you enjoy, songs you sing; deep breaths you take, kisses from loved ones. Think about how your lips and tongue help you articulate your truth. Send gratitude to your mouth for its many vital functions.

Bring awareness to your nose. Think of all the scents that you get to smell. Imagine the aroma of fresh baked bread, seasonal flowers, rainstorms, incense. If you are a yogi, think of ujjayi pranayama, or victorious breath. Send gratitude to your nose for allowing you to breathe and for helping you smell all things accurately.

Bring awareness to your skin. Think of how your skin protects your entire body, from the bottom of your feet to the top of your head. Recognize how your skin allows you to feel sensations of warmth and cold, safety and danger, pain and pleasure. Send gratitude to your skin for encompassing the entirety of who you are.

With awareness and gratitude for your senses and your entire body, in addition to your brain and all your glands, take an inhale; exhale, and release awareness from your senses and your entire body. Remain at rest for the next few minutes or more. Contemplate the congruity of your thoughts-words-actions; mind-body-spirit; past-present-future.

When you are ready, initiate gentle movements: Wiggle your toes and circle your ankles; wiggle your fingers and circle your wrists. Stretch your legs and arms. If you are lying down, rise up to sit. Bring your hands together at your heart to recall and reaffirm your intention or affirmation. Find gratitude for your efforts to reinforce recovery through examination and application of congruency. Inhale, and fill your body with breath; exhale, and return fully to the present moment.

18

Commitment

To understand how the principle of commitment supports recovery, let's first examine three common categories of commitments, how they are formed, and how they require personal attention, time, energy, and other resources to be properly fulfilled. Let's also consider how these types of commitments enhance our mental fitness, emotional sobriety, and physical health, which in turn contribute to our recovery and benefit the lives of all those around us.

CHOSEN COMMITMENTS

This category includes our vocation or employment, marriage and similar partnerships, and religious vows. Before commitments like these are made, we ought to think about how they will influence all aspects of our lives. We should be certain we are prepared to enfold the central elements of these commitments—such as responsibility, fidelity, and dedication—into all our thought processes if we are to know personal homeostasis and contribute to the well-being of others.

NECESSARY COMMITMENTS

This category includes things that sustain existence such as eating, sleeping, and maintaining personal hygiene or cleanliness. For example, when hungry or dehydrated, we can choose to eat healthy foods and drink clean water to nourish and replenish the body. When tired, we can sleep to give the mind, heart, and body rest. When in need of a shower or bath, we can cleanse the outer body to remove impurities; when toxins pervade the inner body, we can fast or partake in related activities to detoxify the organs.

SERVICE COMMITMENTS

This category includes activities like volunteering and assisting others in various altruistic and compassionate ways. For example, if a local organization is hosting a fundraiser, we can offer our time and resources to support the event. If a friend is moving from one home to another, we can organize their belongings and pack or unload boxes. If families in our neighborhood need help getting their children to school, we can participate in a car pool.

Most people can relate to these three types of commitments as foundational components of a civilized and contented human life. Regular adherence to these commitments will safely guide us through a multitude of difficulties that arise throughout everyday situations. However, if those of us who suffer from addictions and equivalent afflictions don't establish and maintain a commitment to recovery foremost among all others, every facet of our lives is placed at risk of serious and rapid disintegration.

COMMITMENT TO RECOVERY

This is a commitment we make to live a consecrated life. It is to allow the beauty of our highest self to emerge from the center of our being. It is to uphold a sacred promise to our mind, body, and spirit to no longer harm or jeopardize the precious human existence we have been given. It is how we express gratitude for being released from the bondage of active addiction. It is how our endeavors are substantiated by clear-minded thinking and disciplined action.

When commitment to recovery is not placed above all other commitments, those things we claim to hold dear—such as loving relationships, career successes, and good health—will no longer be reinforced by the attention and security of an active program of recovery. Without commitment to recovery as our primary objective and continual observance of practices that preserve it, we lose freedom of choice. We become disinterested in self-care. We ignore appeals to be helpful to others. We abandon religious vows and secular obligations. Our best efforts as parents, employees, and neighbors grow lackluster and insufficient. Friendships deteriorate. We no longer feel part of society. Our moral compass spins. The integrity of our sobriety wanes. Our ability to think, say, or do what we inherently know to be good and true withers and evaporates. Ultimately, if recovery and the personal routines that preserve it are not prioritized to the utmost among all our obligations and concerns, every category of our inner and outer lives regresses or completely dissolves until recovery *is* established as our chief commitment.

STEADFASTNESS AND COMMITMENT TO RECOVERY

Within the yogic tradition, the Sanskrit term *sthairyam* denotes steadfastness. Etymologically, this word can also be defined as "steadiness," "firmness," or "stability," since the root *stha* expresses an enduring capacity "to take up a station or position" and "to continue in any action or condition."

Sthairyam is necessary upon any path to recovery. It allows us to face all challenges throughout our lives. It prepares us to be cautious and practical when confronted by people, places, or things that threaten our sanity or sobriety. It emboldens us to accurately identify personal liabilities and transform them into assets. It helps us recognize and avoid enticements that weaken our resolve to achieve goals.

Addiction is a nefarious opportunist. It knows how to lure victims away from rituals and defenses that fortify recovery. It belittles our determination so that we feel lost and disoriented. It employs doubt, depression, and procrastination to distract us. It depends upon the influences of lust and shame to suspend our attempts to remain poised. It promises prestige, wealth, and power since pursuit of these fixations leads to personal dissatisfaction, which promotes vacillation and indifference. It also capitalizes on the relationship between insecurity and pride so that mental and emotional breakdowns occur instead of physical and spiritual breakthroughs.

Addiction knows our likes and dislikes, fears and jealousies, attachments and resentments. It uses our past, present, and future weaknesses against us. It exploits all of these concepts and more to destabilize us when and where we least expect confrontation. It is eternally committed to the destruction of every department of our lives until we succumb to its temptations.

Without sthairyam as part of our recovery, we become vulnerable when addiction casts its nets of darkness over us from behind the facade of its myriad disguises. If we are not actively working a program of recovery, we become absent-minded and apathetic. Our ability and willingness to protect ourselves declines, and we become complacent. Our beneficial practices are deprioritized or abandoned, and we are unable to strengthen or sustain recovery. Addiction then targets and penetrates all unguarded areas of our lives until its terrors are instilled within our mind and allegiance is induced from our body.

LET'S MAKE THIS PERSONAL

A commitment to recovery requires certain practices and protections. Read the following questions and write down your answers. Share your thoughts with friends in recovery or a supportive peer group. Discuss areas within your life that can be modified to enhance a commitment to recovery.

What do you do each day to preserve the quality of your recovery? Do you have a regular routine? Is your day structured so that recovery takes precedence? Which of your daily activities strengthen your commitment to recovery? Which of your everyday pursuits or pastimes weaken your commitment to recovery?

What tempts you to stray from recovery practices or exercises? Can you explore ways to keep current practices fresh and exciting? Can you amend or remove activities that no longer positively affect your recovery? Can you add a new activity or mode of inspiration to improve your recovery? Can you recommit to a former custom you have abandoned?

Do you find yourself chasing after certain cravings or sensual pleasures? Do you distract yourself with outer stimuli to avoid being in the reality of now? Where in your day are you not making good use of your time? When in your day are you able or unable to be present with yourself and others?

Do egoism, pride, or prejudice dissuade you from attending twelve-step meetings or similar gatherings where recovery is the central point of focus? Are you accountable to others in regard to keeping your commitment to recovery? Do you regularly offer and receive support from others in recovery? Are you remaining teachable, humble, open-minded, and willing to grow as you continue your recovery journey?

19

Concentration

Concentration in recovery means fixing our attention on a particular object or subject to inspire change. It is applying intense focus and singularly-directed energy into or toward a specific area for desired and useful purposes. It means inviting the mind to abide in a state of inner stillness so that we can receive intuitive thoughts. It is exploring deeper, expansive realms within our consciousness so we can interpret divine guidance. Ultimately it is how we channel individual and universal powers to induce all forms of enlightenment.

Imagine a boy holding a magnifying glass outside to catch sunlight within the convex lens of his instrument. If he positions his arm accordingly and directs sunshine through the glass onto a sheet of paper on the ground and he remains poised and patient and does not allow his mind to wander nor his hand to waver, he may eventually see smoke appear at the spot where the sunbeam hits the paper. If conditions are right, he may also welcome a little flame within the same area.

This process of transformation exemplifies the inseparability of effort and faith and how they mutually engender completeness of concentration to elicit extraordinary results. As much as the boy may try to set the paper aflame on his own power, it will not happen. He needs both personal determination and the contribution of a higher source of energy to create fire. If he is to alter his personal circumstances and outer surroundings, he must combine human, finite strengths and rudimentary tools with universal, infinite powers and perfected resources. If he initiates and preserves an alliance between these relative and absolute energies, he will learn that anything is possible with the right balance of knowledge, dedication, and practice. He will learn the dynamic and necessary interplay of application and surrender. He will learn that he will never need to face any challenges alone. He will also learn that when concentration is properly composed, he can change every aspect of his life and the world in which he lives.

This example describes how concentration ought to be applied within the lives of people in recovery. We must recognize that under our own power we can't personally metamorphose the entirety of any addiction. We must be convinced that no amount of individualized effort can transmute perverse cravings and degenerative habits into emancipation unless accompanied by the support of an unlimited source of power. We must re-member that addiction is a dark, otherworldly force comprising unfathomable and multilayered features. Thus, we can't expect victory over addiction if we employ unaided mental concentration to combat its irrationality—a rational mind is no match for the unpredictability of addiction nor its inhumane assaults.

To rise above the overwhelming dynamism of addiction, we must summon the strength of supernatural resources and forge sacred partnerships. Our concentration must be multidimensional, higher-powered, and imbued with a customized spiritual component to successfully support all stages of recovery. And since spiritual awareness is without borders and the spiritual dimension itself can't be calculated, the depths and efficacy of spiritualized concentration are immeasurable. As a result, no task in recovery becomes too difficult and no situation in life is unmanageable—so long as we continue to foster relationships with chosen spiritual and similarly special entities through daily and reverential acts of recognition.

FAITH AND CONCENTRATION

Yogic scriptures avow that *shraddha*, or faith, is necessary if we are to intuit our svadharma, or personal purpose, and ascertain how to successfully align mental and spiritual energies to fulfill it. The word *shraddha* comes from two Sanskrit words: *shrat*, which means "truth" or "faithfulness," and *dha*, which can be interpreted as "to direct one's mind toward."

Shraddha allows us to glimpse the inmost actuality of who we are and the absoluteness and significance of our unique existence. It gives us vision and sustains our volition. It protects us as we encounter obstacles upon the trajectory of our path as sentient beings. It comforts and heartens all spiritualists seeking truth; yogis beholding *Prema*, or divine love; worshippers of God; humanists embracing the majesty of Mother Earth; secularists acknowledging the indelibility of nature or the universe; and all persons contemplating relationships with Spirit, Source, and equivalent forms of infinite intelligence.

Shraddha elevates the mind and body beyond everyday thought and action. When the mind is directed onto itself in search of truth, what is revealed can only be enlightened instruction. Armed with such inner knowing, our mentality becomes rightly concentrated and can be directed outwardly with devotion and single-pointedness. Our concentration will then reflect internal convictions and reinforce inmost truths while simultaneously penetrating worthy subjects of contemplation.

Without shraddha, our attention becomes scattered. We squander time investigating things that do not reflect our true values or contribute to the evolution of our purpose. When we spend time deliberating about things not aligned with our personal understandings of truth, love, God, and comparable concepts, the mind becomes fatigued and listless and the body weakens and grows susceptible to temptations.

If shraddha is to successfully shape concentration, we must examine how we spend our time and what we think about most often. We must look at where our energies are expended and how they are allotted or compartmentalized. And we must consciously withdraw attentiveness and allegiance from incorrect and inappropriate objectives that destabilize the psyche and impede spiritual development and redirect our focus toward matters that uplift our mentality and deepen spiritual acuity.

LET'S MAKE THIS PERSONAL

Read the following questions and answer them to the best of your ability. Look for patterns within areas of your life where your strengths may be depleted, your attention may be fragmented, and your energy may be misdirected. Look for where you may struggle to accomplish things independently. Look for where you may be able to nurture conviction and invite collaboration.

What do your thoughts dwell on most often? A specific person or group of people? A certain place or institution? A particular thing or possession? An unhealthy obsession or dependence? Regrets about the past or anxieties about the future? What is the quality of your attention in regard to any of these things?

What are your interests throughout the day? Do they contain a balance of intelligence and action? Are they healthy, inspiring, and helpful to you and others? Do they reinforce your sense of purpose?

Are you consciously invested in the daily upkeep of your recovery? Are you interested in all aspects of recovery—mental, emotional, physical, and spiritual? What does recovery bring to your life? What do you bring to your recovery?

How are you faithful to your innermost self? Whom or what do you call upon for help when lost or disillusioned? Where do you place your trust when you encounter personal problems? Do you believe a higher power can help you achieve things that you can't accomplish on your own?

PRACTICING CONCENTRATION

The following breathing meditation can be utilized to generate concentration. Choose a location that encourages *ekagrata*, or single-pointed focus. Candles, incense, or sage can be lit to create sacred space. An altar can be prepared with flowers, photos, or statues of deities. Silence is an ideal condition to receive the benefits of this practice.

Begin in a cross-legged seated position. Sit so your spine remains upright. If sitting cross-legged is not possible, a chair can be used, or lie on your back. Cushions and folded blankets can provide support for specific areas of your body, if needed.

Bring awareness to your in-breath and out-breath. Distinguish the inhale, exhale, and space between breaths. Breathe consciously; notice how focusing on the breath calms your mind. The breath is prana, or life force, and flows throughout thousands of nadis, or channels, within the body. Take a moment to send gratitude to your breath for vitalizing your mind, body, and spirit.

Take a deep inhale; allow the exhale to anchor your mind into the present moment.

Take a deep inhale; allow the exhale to root your consciousness in the here and now.

Take a deep inhale; allow the exhale to create sound as prayer.

Take a deep inhale and feel the density of your physical body; allow the exhale to create space to accept things as they are in the reality of now.

Take a deep inhale; on the exhale, feel contact with the earth.

Take a deep inhale; on the exhale, relax your physical body.

Take a deep inhale; on the exhale, release preconceived notions regarding meditation.

Take a deep inhale; on the exhale, allow this meditation to be a courageous exploration of your mind, body, and spirit.

Take a deep inhale; on the exhale, open your eyes.

Take a deep inhale; and on the exhale, smile.

20

Meditation

Meditation can be likened to a raft that brings us to the other shore of enlightenment. It bridges various states of consciousness within the reality of now to deliver us from fear to love, anger to calm, and stagnation to transformation. It is an introspective and personal journey that allows us to glimpse who and what we truly are through honest self-assessment of current mental formations.

Meditation offers myriad opportunities for us to analyze what lies upon the surface and within the peripheries and depths of the human mind. When such findings are analyzed with proper discernment and dispassionate observation, we come to know our natural or resting state as neutral—if we can accept things as they are in the here and now. Thus, meditation reveals the health of our mentality and emotionality in correlation with our spirituality as we explore energetic layers throughout the entirety of the body and encounter the effulgence of the innermost spirit or soul.

Meditation helps all seekers detect the duality of our citizenship within the ultimate dimension or vertical plane of existence and the historical dimension or horizontal plane of existence. Through physical solidity and mental stability cultivated in meditation, we can explore and absorb insights contained within these interdependent realms and safely integrate our discoveries within the certitude and security of the present moment.

Meditation and its benefits are available to anyone who chooses to practice. All pursuers of truth and serenity, stillness and silence, balance and peace—regardless of creed, caste, race, or sex—can meditate and receive innumerable holistic rewards. All human beings can come home to themselves with present-moment awareness in meditation and perceive the certainties of existence, understand the mysteries of the cosmos, and touch the many miracles of mindfulness that include healing, wellness, and recovery.

PRACTICING MEDITATION

Meditation styles and techniques vary with regard to their histories and methodologies. Many religious and spiritual practices were created and systematized thousands of years ago to quiet the mind and connect seekers to God or a supreme reality, but these methods are just as effective now as when they originated. Modern, secular forms of evidence-based meditation have been scientifically proven to alleviate various symptoms of suffering and are presently utilized in clinical and therapeutic settings to address stress reduction, trauma resolution, and addiction treatment. Contemporary and intuitive forms of meditation can be organic, creative hybrids of past and present traditions and include ecstatic dance and similar movement-based expression; flower-arranging, leaf-raking, earth-touching, and other nature-oriented action; abstract painting, mandala drawing, and personalized artistic endeavors; and mantra chanting or likewise incantation observances to cultivate and receive blessings for things such as protection, abundance, and wisdom.

Possibilities for meditation are endless since each individual practitioner is unique and possesses personal inclinations about what may be enjoyed or preferred. Therefore, meditators ought to select beneficial practices that suit their individual temperaments and the modes or processes that meet their current needs. Meditators can also profit from remaining open-minded and exploring unfamiliar practices that can complement regular routines and expand spiritual viewpoints.

Meditation for people in recovery is no different from meditation for others who don't suffer from dependences. However, many people in recovery tend to share common mental peculiarities, emotional sensitivities, physical cravings, and spiritual deficiencies that don't typically afflict those without compulsive and despondent constitutions, chemically induced fixations, and related attachment-based issues. Therefore, those in recovery may wish to consider the following suggestions and yogic guiding principles to create and maintain a meditation practice that can neutralize the predictable, particular, and penetrative effects of addiction.

Find a Quiet and Clean Location

Addiction thrives within chaos and clutter. It loves noise and distractions. It prefers to attack people in active addiction or those in recovery at locations where our attention is scattered or intermittent.

When we become unfocused and discombobulated, we can't perceive our innermost truth; consequently, obsessive and addictive thinking becomes our default mode of cognition. However, when safe, sacred spaces are created for solitude and meditation, the collective energies of *mauna*, or silence, and saucha, or purity, protect all meditators and our practices can become an effective, powerful means to turn our attention inward to accurately sense and interpret the clarity and wisdom of our highest self.

Find a Comfortable Position and Cultivate Stillness

Addiction can hardly overtake a truly stable person; thus, it targets and assails those who are unable to regularly remain mentally and bodily still. Within contemporary yogic phraseology, the Sanskrit term *asana* is typically defined as "pose" or "posture"; however, another rendering of this ancient term is "seat" since the true purpose of asana is to position the body in a manner by which the complementary qualities of *sthira*, or steadiness, and *sukha*, or ease, are harmonious so that the supreme inner work of meditation can transpire.

When the body is composed and relaxed, the mind can actively employ concentration, contemplation, and correlated techniques to reach a heightened state of consciousness known as *samadhi*, or union with the divine. The mind can't achieve autonomy or emancipation unless the body can disregard the energy of carnal urges and other obsessions of the flesh. It is only through the negation of physical rigidity and restlessness that individual consciousness can unify with universal consciousness in meditation. And it is only when the outer body settles that *buddhi*, or the awakened aspect of the inner mind, can clearly perceive its inherent luminescence.

Close Your Eyes

Addiction does not wish for meditators to know that peace and harmony are eternally available in the present moment. Therefore, it exploits *caksurvijnana*, or eye consciousness, to divert our attention into the past or future through manipulation of visual perceptions that can invoke emotions, memories, and projections.

When people, places, and things are optically recognized as familiar, yogic philosophy asserts that personal inferences in relation to each object of perception arise within the mind of the viewer; it is these undertones that disturb our inhabiting the reality of now as the mind becomes preoccupied with flashbacks, uncertainties, expectations, and other obscurations. Contrarily, when pratyahara, or withdrawal of the senses, is practiced through closing our two physical eyes, outer distractions—positive, negative, or otherwise—are eliminated, and meditators can draw upon the impartiality of mystical insights from the ajna chakra, or third-eye center, rather than rely on the subjectivity of outer visualization from the two physical eyes.

Breathe with Awareness

Addiction strives to occupy the mind with endless cycles of morbid reflections on unwholesome desires. It destabilizes all healthy thought patterns with frequent transfusions of negativity, busyness, and ruination. It leaves people in recovery constantly deliberating causes and effects of darkness and death so the mind becomes inert and insane, and eventually will lead the body toward intoxication.

Within the yogic tradition, the breath is regarded as prana, or life force. When attention is brought to the in-breath and out-breath, our mental capacities focus on something animate, life-affirming, and positive; something illuminating, natural, and rhythmic; something that devotedly and reassuringly directs us from one transformational moment to the next within the reality of now.

Mindful breathing sustains and steadies the mind; it nourishes and strengthens the body; and it establishes and maintains conscious contact with the spirit. Every human being has breath in their body; therefore, anyone in recovery can bring awareness to the inhale and exhale to counteract the psychological brutalities and other mental deceptions and morbidities of addiction.

A Guided Meditation for Recovery

Below is a guided meditation that encompasses and elaborates upon the concepts and principles above. Utilize this script in any manner that works best for you. For example, you could read or record the words verbatim and meditate as outlined. You could also personalize these suggestions to supplement your regular practice methods. Or you could gather with others in recovery and one person could lead the group through this meditation.

Before you begin, consider setting a sankalpa, or intention, for something you wish to achieve from this meditation. Also, you may light a candle or stick of incense and recite a favorite prayer, mantra, or chant that can protect or guide you through this journey. Pause as necessary to reflect upon your experiences, embrace emotions and memories as they arise, and perhaps record your insights into a journal. Ultimately, allow this meditation to nourish your mind and body in the present moment so that you can touch the wellspring of calm, balance, and peace forever available within your heart.

Find a quiet, safe space. Find a comfortable seat or position and begin to settle in. Close your eyes and begin to relax your body. Take a deep inhale; exhale and let it go. Again, take a deep inhale; exhale and let it go. One last time, take a deep inhale; exhale and let it go.

Allow gravity to befriend you as you continue to relax your body. Begin to feel the earth beneath you. Recognize its qualities of steadiness, stability, solidity. Know that the earth is our foundation. Feel a sense of groundedness beneath you. Know that the earth will not drop you in this moment, you will not fall in this moment, you will not be abandoned in this moment, you will not be rejected in this moment. Know that you will be held and supported during this meditation, you will be lifted above the heaviness and density of addiction during this meditation, you will feel the lightness and levity of recovery during this meditation. Let all of these ideas permeate your mind and heart for the next few moments in silence as you continue to breathe consciously and allow awareness of your breath to anchor your mind in the here and now.

Allow the earth to truly absorb the heaviness of your life, the density of your arms and legs, the weight of the world that you may be carrying on your shoulders. Release burdens, worries, or responsibilities that may currently be on your mind or within your heart. Release attachments to people, places, and things that may hold you back from being your highest self in this moment. Release old ideas, conditioned behaviors, and limiting beliefs that do not serve the positive development of your recovery today. For the next few moments, rest in silence as you continue to breathe consciously and allow the earth to support and hold you throughout this healing and transformative process.

Begin to bring awareness back to the present moment. Inhale and feel the lightness of your being, the weightlessness of life, the ease and buoyancy of recovery. Exhale and cultivate gratitude for the present moment; honor your courage and determination; embrace the miracle of recovery.

Begin to bring awareness back to your physical body. Inhale and feel the safety and security of the space around you, the heart of the earth beneath you, the heart of the sky above you. Exhale and feel the spiritual dimension of your heart and know that it holds within it infinite intelligence, immense power, and unconditional love.

Begin to wiggle your fingers and toes; circle your wrists and ankles. Come back fully to the present moment. Inhale and feel harmony within your mind, body, and spirit. Exhale and know that your life is purposeful and you are a miracle. When you are ready to begin your day anew, gently blink your eyes open.

21

Compassion

Compassion in recovery is depending on one another for individual and collective healing, reciprocal growth, and universal transformation. It is becoming intimate with personal sufferings and their respective solutions so that we can recognize similar pains within the minds and hearts of others in order to console such persons in need. It is to comprehend that addictions and related problems are part of a communal spiritual curriculum in which emotional, mental, and physical causes of disharmony are identified and remedied through fellowship with those in recovery, in addition to brotherhood and sisterhood with people in all areas of our lives.

Compassion in recovery begins with oneself if it is to be authentic and effective. When its three foundational components of self-acceptance, self-forgiveness, and self-love are implemented within a program of action, a boundless capacity to empathize with others is forged in our consciousness. This state of inner disarmament can then express itself benevolently throughout our relations with all people, places, and things.

Let's examine the essentials of self-acceptance, self-forgiveness, and self-love to see how these three concepts conjoin with yogic principles and practices to help us overcome personal defects, complexes, and neuroses so that we can better serve others; inspire us to make peace with inner demons so that we can emancipate others from mental and emotional distress; and encourage us to venerate our existence so that we can help others honor the miracle of life.

SELF-ACCEPTANCE

If we don't accept the facts of our lives, we can't transmute personal afflictions; our thought processes remain in a perpetual state of degeneration; and our tolerance for the shortcomings of others will be inadequate. When individual deficiencies are neglected throughout recovery, our mindset will be influenced by denial, ignorance, and pride; our capacity for sympathy will be weak; and we will be incapable of offering kindness to the world. If self-acceptance is not regularly practiced in all areas of life, we can't overcome pain related to fear of the unknown, withstand the implications of nagging doubts and hesitancies, or be helpful to anyone who suffers from confusion, pessimism, and embarrassment.

Gentleness is the key to mastering self-acceptance so that vanity, spitefulness, and complacency can't impede the accumulation and assimilation of positive, negative, and neutral truths nor hinder the natural unfolding of our spiritual development. Therefore, we must never blame or judge ourselves for where we are in life or begrudge how we may have arrived at this moment. We must not pity ourselves for things we have done or resent what may have been done to us. We should not attach meaning to what we choose to accept or analyze the ramifications of our acknowledgments.

When personal truths are thus recognized rather than repudiated, we discover *upeksha*, or equanimity, within oneself as a state of inclusiveness inherent in the heart of every human being. When such an experiential basis of understanding is acquired, inner dissonances cease to disturb our mentality and emotive whirlwinds no longer disorient our natural proclivities toward altruistic thought and action. Armed with such pragmatic wisdom, we can heal personal wounds and compassionately attend to mutual misfortunes within the minds and hearts of others.

Upeksha can be cultivated by meditating on the nature of suffering as an inalienable truth within the lives of all human beings. The following declarations nourish the seed of *karuna*, or compassion, within our consciousness so that upeksha can support our efforts to accept the dualism of suffering and happiness.

Practicing Self-Acceptance

Find a comfortable, seated position. Take three conscious breaths to anchor your awareness in the reality of now. Silently repeat the sentences below or read them aloud. Meditate on the words and allow their meaning to suffuse your heart with compassion for yourself and all human beings.

May I make peace with my sufferings and learn from my mistakes.

May I remember that I am human and to err is part of my nature.

May I remember that my soul is divine, thus transcendence is my birthright.

May compassion arise within me today as I live in harmony with all aspects of my humanity and my divinity.

SELF-FORGIVENESS

Guilt, regret, and similar vulnerabilities must be purged from our intellect if we are to offer leniency to others. We can't extend tenderness if our spirit is saddled by personal grievances, grudges, and other things left unprocessed or neglected. When we remain unforgiving toward ourselves, our insecurities project outwardly and prevent us from intuiting the inmost essence of goodness within others. If we continue to suffer from personal brokenness or perpetual culpability throughout recovery, openheartedness can't be externally shared nor can a suitable replacement be offered while the mind remains impure.

We must offer ourselves mercy in recovery if self-forgiveness is to be a realistic and fundamental element of compassion. Without an inward allowance of charity for any unwholesome or unskillful things we have thought, spoken, or done in the past, our temperament will remain blighted by remorse and delusiveness. Our morality will be undermined by pangs of shame and sorrow. Malevolence will envelop our conscience. We will feel indignant toward ourselves. We will be shortsighted about our present motives and dread the consequences of our actions.

Without the integration of mercy as a method for working with personal transgressions in recovery, we will also not look kindly on the wrongdoings of others in active addiction. We will lack sympathy for friends who have had a lapse in judgment. We will perceive the errors and weaknesses of our neighbors as immoral. We will be critical and callous in regard to the daily happenings of colleagues in the workplace. We will feel disingenuous among spiritual companions. We will withdraw affection and attention from those we love at home.

When we recognize *kshama*, or forbearance, in recovery as a means to liberate ourselves from the burdens that are overwhelming our perspective, we can offer amnesty to ourselves and subsequently to all beings. Kshama helps us exonerate unforgivable moments within our lives through the cultivation of patience and understanding in regard to the various stages of our spiritual development. Kshama rescues us from psychological prisons of our own making as it emboldens us to stop reliving deplorable memories or revisiting their respective repercussions. Kshama also allows us to learn the causes, conditions, and consequences of our errors so that we can compassionately assist others who may be crippled beneath the weight of their mistakes.

Kshama can be developed by consciously examining our unresolved emotions and holistically healing areas of the body where they reside. *Supta baddha-konasana*, or reclining bound-angle pose, opens the hips and stretches the thighs and inner groin. This posture helps us realize forgiveness through the attainments of physical spaciousness and relaxation, emotional vulnerability and sincerity, mental stability and composure, spiritual awareness and sanctuary.

Practicing Self-Forgiveness

Find a level, safe space on the ground and have pillows and blankets nearby. Sit upright on a yoga mat and bring the soles of your feet together. Place pillows or blankets beneath your knees so that the knees are supported comfortably. Place pillows or blankets behind you on the mat and lie down upon them so that your back and body are comfortable. Set a pillow or blanket beneath your head so that your head is comfortable. Rest your arms alongside your body atop any extra pillows and blankets so that your arms are comfortable.

Relax the weight of your body and settle in to your position. Begin to breathe deeply; recognize the rise and fall of your abdomen with each inhale and exhale. Place your right hand over your belly and your left hand over your heart; feel the volume of the breath moving beneath your hands. Continue to breathe deeply and consciously. Allow your knees to be heavy. Allow the space across your chest to broaden. Allow your shoulders to relax. Allow your elbows to rest on the ground or on pillows.

With your in-breath, call to mind a grudge, grievance, or something you have not forgiven within yourself. With your out-breath, release that which no longer serves you. Repeat this process as needed to let go of specific instances of anger, guilt, shame, resentment, and similar emotions. Remember that your breath is with you and guiding you. It is purifying your mind, body, and spirit. It is delivering you to the other shore of liberation. It is your innermost teacher. It is leading you home to your heart where compassion resides.

To end this practice, bring your hands to your outer knees

and draw them inward. Wrap your arms around your shins and give yourself a hug. Roll onto either side of your body and pause to reflect on your experience. Sit up tall and bring your hands together at your heart. Lower your chin toward your chest and bow into yourself. Acknowledge the space, freedom, forgiveness, and compassion you have cultivated within your mind, heart, body, and spirit.

SELF-LOVE

When our self-regard is hateful or unkind, our perspective will be governed by hostility, weariness, and indecisiveness, and we will be unable to effectively offer patience, understanding, or consolation to others. Without love in our hearts for ourselves, self-respect will be lacking in our disposition, and we will be unable to honor our feelings or commiserate with the emotions of others. Without conscious awareness of love as a guiding force in our recovery, we will not be able to convert our past or current pain into purposefulness or support this transformational process within the lives of those who suffer from addictions and other problems.

When we can't love ourselves, our self-valuation will be poor, and we will wrongly identify personal assets as liabilities. For example, we will lack confidence in our natural talents and learned skills. We will be unable to trust our beliefs or sensory impressions. We will doubt the validity of our heartfelt opinions and experiences. We will abandon our established hopes and dreams. We will forsake our spiritual practices and recovery principles.

If self-loathing completely shrouds our perception, we will

not comprehend that love infuses our thoughts, words, and actions with sincerity and efficacy when we endeavor to minister to others in need. We will not recognize that love transmutes our selfishness into selflessness, and our self-centeredness into other-centeredness, thus making us useful instruments for bringing peace, calm, balance, and compassion to others. We will not fathom that love inspires us when we share our personal experience, strength, and hope with others at a twelve-step meeting or similar gathering in the hopes that all persons present can avoid the hardships of active addiction.

Practicing Self-Love

The yogic mantra *Aham Prema*, which can be translated as "I Am Love," remedies predispositions toward all thoughts and actions of self-hatred. Recitation of this mantra opens, heals, and harmonizes the mind and heart. This eternal, spiritual truth affirms that our present human incarnation is a precious manifestation of unbounded, unparalleled, and undividable love and that our collective purpose as human beings is to freely and compassionately give and receive that which heals, transforms, and sustains us.

Stand or sit comfortably in front of a mirror. Take a few moments to consider the inner child within you who may have needed affection, understanding, or a sense of security. Embrace the teenager within you who may have needed friendship, happiness, or spiritual guidance. Recognize the adult within you who may have needed empathy, comfort, and a sense of belonging. Connect with the person you are today and offer every aspect of yourself unconditional love and compassion in the here and now.

Aham Prema—or "I Am Love"—can now be chanted 108 times to correspond with each of the nadis, or energetic channels, which surround the heart. You can look into the mirror as you chant or close your eyes to internalize your practice. Place your hands at your heart or in your lap. Each time the mantra is repeated, feel the synchronization of love and compassion within your heart. Feel your vision being renewed so that you will see yourself and all living beings with eyes of compassion. Feel your ears being attuned so that you will hear the cries of the world and be able to respond in a compassionate manner. Feel your language being enhanced so that your words will comfort and heal the suffering of others. Feel your body being strengthened so that you can lift up those who have fallen down. Finally, feel every cell in your body being infused by the incomparable and infinite energies of love in all forms, including human, divine, and universal.

22

Mindfulness

Mindfulness is the ability to direct our awareness and hold our attention upon a specific, chosen area or topic of interest. It is a means to focus and concentrate on whatever we are doing in the present moment so that our thoughts, words, and actions will be intentional and constructive. It is a way to honor the mind, body, and spirit since mindfulness allows us to properly utilize our time and energy to treasure the many miracles of life and offer the fruits of these experiences to others.

When mindfulness is developed and strengthened as a daily practice and its features are integrated into recovery, we can better understand our mental investigations, emotional quandaries, and metaphysical musings. We can discover and heal root causes that have contributed to the manifestation of our disease or addiction.

We can visualize and actualize a path that leads away from trauma or darkness toward awakening and freedom.

Mindfulness can't be achieved, however, if the mind and body are under the influence of alcohol, drugs, or addictive behaviors. Sobriety is necessary if we are to successfully practice mindfulness in recovery; thus, we must refrain from ingesting toxins or stimulants that alter our mental state and stop behaving in ways that negatively influence our body so that rational thoughts and wholesome actions can support mindfulness practices.

Similarly, it is challenging to be mindful if our consciousness is under the influence of things like fear, anger, indecision, insecurity, and jealousy. Therefore, we must attempt to abstain from thinking or acting in ways that produce these and similar feelings and emotions. For instance, we can take a break from ruminating about past mistakes or future concerns and avoid interacting with others in situations where we know our inner hostilities and resentments may be roused.

Mindfulness can be cultivated at any time of day, anywhere in the world, by anyone who chooses to receive its rewards. For example, we can focus on the length of our next inhale and the depth of the following exhale. We can notice our footsteps the next time we walk from one spot to another. We can look at the shapes and colors of leaves on the next tree that we see. Teeth-brushing, dish-washing, and vegetable-cutting are additional examples of how any moment can be an opportunity to practice mindfulness and experience its benefits, which include stress reduction, mood stabilization, and present-moment awareness.

With so many options to generate mindfulness, those in recovery can prioritize certain theories and practices in order to create and sustain a purposeful life of abstinence and contentment. Foremost, we ought to become aware of the negative and unwholesome ways toxins of all kinds are consumed so that harmful or conditioned patterns that lead to dependences can be eliminated. Next, we must realize that our thoughts, speech, and actions are directly influenced by many nutriments, which in turn affect the health and unity of the mind, body, and spirit. Last, we should make good use of the insights revealed during individual and collective mindfulness practices so that personal endeavors and interpersonal relations exemplify and honor our universality and interconnectedness with all living things.

MINDFULNESS OF CONSUMPTION

Within the yogic tradition, there are many forms of *ahara*, or food, recognized as the principal means to nourish the totality of our existence. Although this teaching is thousands of years old, it is quite relevant today as it provides an enduring guideline for mindfulness in consumption. For those in recovery, two aharas are of utmost concern if we wish to remain healthy and eliminate the possibility of relapse and other types of regressions that prohibit proper nourishment, psychological and physiological uniformity, and long-term recovery. These are edible foods and sensory impressions.

Let's explore these two aharas from a modern and universal standpoint to see how to make informed, mindful choices about what we ingest or absorb each day. Let's investigate various sources of nutriments to discover how they affect our constitution, behavior, and perspective so that we can properly feed our mental, emotional, physical, and spiritual health. Let's determine practical ways to deal with unhealthy cravings so that we can amend unmindful or compulsive patterns of consumption. And let's consider integrating beneficial solutions discovered within these processes alongside positive, effective components that comprise our daily dietary and recovery regimens.

Edible Foods

Nutrition can often be overlooked as an essential element when a person is attempting to get clean or sober since other health concerns, such as internal bleeding or possible organ failure, may be more prominent and require immediate attention during this time. However, when physical stabilization is achieved and mental equilibrium is attained, we must become mindful of how edible foods are consumed and how our diet helps or hinders the quality of our health and happiness in recovery.

In recovery, we can eat in ways that nourish both our body and our conscience. We can stabilize the mind and gladden the heart by consuming foods in a way that accords with our personal beliefs. For example, if a person professes to love animals, they can eat a vegetarian or vegan diet so that their dietary choices will not contribute to the harming of animals. If another person wants to protect the planet, they can eat in ways that help reverse land degradation, climate change, air or water pollution, and other ecosystem threats. If a group aspires to create a sustainable future for forthcoming generations, they can opt to use recyclable utensils, cups, and plates in addition to reusable bottles and containers.

Throughout recovery, we can strive to become knowledgeable about what is in the foods we eat, where our foods are grown, and how our foods are produced and packaged. We can learn to read labels on food items and figure out how to research the origins of all ingredients. We can be mindful about eating foods that have been artificially or genetically modified or exposed to synthetic and potentially harmful pesticides. We can also be wary if we decide to ingest stimulants such as caffeine, sugar, and nicotine, since regular consumption of products like these may trigger old, addictive mental patterns that can be troublesome for recovered alcoholics or addicts.

When we become cognizant of how edible nutriments affect the individual functionality and collective solidarity of the mind, body, and spirit, we can make a vow to protect the sanctity of our health and recovery by eating in moderation and ingesting only what is nutritious, energizing, healing, and congruent with personal values and recovery principles.

LET'S MAKE THIS PERSONAL

Do you feel that you eat in a healthy way? Do you eat meals on a regular schedule? Do you eat or snack at odd or random times? Do you eat when you are not hungry? Do you eat as a way to avoid emotional pain or suffering? Do you know where your food comes from? Do you know what is in your food? Do you know how your food is prepared or produced? Do you express gratitude for your meals and the means by which you receive food? Do your dietary choices align with your recovery and lifestyle principles?

Sensory Impressions

A prominent hallmark of personal recovery is autonomy. When the mind is no longer dominated by the impulses of active addictions and we have recovered from mental enslavement associated with dependences, in addition to the physical attachment and spiritual deterioration that accompanies misguided desires, lustful cravings, and harmful habits, we are free to make independent choices based on personal likes and dislikes that align with recovery ideologies. When we attain sovereignty after the bondage of disease and its psychic detritus, we can customize our personal and professional lives in a multitude of ways that not only suit productive, preferential tastes but also enhance and support the positive lifestyle choices of friends and others we come in contact with. And when we are in control of all our determinations in recovery, we can consciously select how to nourish our senses with healthy forms of sustenance so that emotional sobriety—which can be considered the pillar of lasting recovery—can be stabilized and continue to remain balanced.

When we absorb sensory inputs, our emotions are affected. Our vitality can be either weakened or strengthened as a result. For example, exposure to violent visual media can stimulate in some people internal tendencies toward aggression, desensitization toward imagined or real displays of violence, and, in some cases, mimicry of what has been viewed. A steady diet of pornography can lead some people to objectify and sexualize others, suffer from delusional or fanatical thinking and unhealthy obsessions or infatuations, and experience the deterioration of their personal morality and physical degradation through pursuit of sensual gratification. A person who views a documentary or biopic about the life and teachings of a revered saint or savior may feel inspired to positively change individual habits, contemplate the intersection of humanity and spirituality, and devote more time and energy toward acts of love and service for others.

And another person who views an animated, child-friendly film with family or friends may feel a sense of wonder, joy, or hope; commonality among loved ones; and genuine affection for all humankind and nature.

If external stimuli can exasperate or enliven internal emotions but we are not mindful of what we consume through our senses, we open ourselves up to whatever emotional perturbations or enhancements come our way to manifest throughout the mind. When such states of fluctuation are ongoing, *citta vrittis*, or mental whirlpools, form within our consciousness, which inhibits our ability to make definitive choices in regard to healthy or unhealthy nutriments. If we remain unmindful of how sensory stimuli initiate changes in our temperament, emotional regulation—which begets emotional sobriety—will be unlikely to manifest.

When we recognize how conscious and unconscious sensory preferences invite positive and negative stimuli into the brain, which in turn, directly influences the emotionality of our thoughts, speech, and actions, we can vow to make intelligent and wholesome choices in regard to what we allow to penetrate our gates of perception—the eyes, ears, nose, mouth, and skin—and only spend our time, energy, and money in accordance with things that nourish our health and recovery.

LET'S MAKE THIS PERSONAL

What types of TV programs, films, or videos do you watch? What kinds of newspapers, magazines, or books do you read? Which websites do you regularly view on the internet? Which applications do you frequently use on your computer or electronic devices? Which radio stations or other listening formats do you utilize to hear music, talks, or teachings? What are the topics and tone of your conversations with others?

How do your choices of sensory stimuli affect you? Are they nourishing? Beneficial? Which emotions or feelings arise within you when you consume your choices of content? How do your preferences affect your mind and temperament? How do your selections nourish your heart and spirit? How do you feel after you consume your chosen forms of media, entertainment, or leisure?

23

Simplicity

When simplicity is taken as a guiding principle within a program of recovery, our thoughts, words, and actions become efficient, timely, and orderly. Simplicity arranges our lives so that our moral propensities, mental energies, physical exertions, and spiritual sensitivities holistically support all aspects of our healing and transformation. It is simplicity that allows us to enjoy whatever we are doing in the present moment—for example, breathing when we are breathing, sitting when we are sitting, walking when we are walking—without a need to think about the past or future, a desire to change anything about our current situation, or a wish that our circumstances should somehow be different.

When simplicity oversees all details of recovery, harmony and freedom become constant companions, and whatever needs to be accomplished is completed in perfect time, without unnecessary deliberation or hesitation. When we simply do whatever is in front of us in any given moment, without bias or individual preference, we no longer suffer from confusion or doubt, and we naturally intuit how to achieve both short- and long-term goals. When we simplify the manner by which we manage personal choices and arrange chores, our lifestyle becomes streamlined, which affords us the time and energy to help others define and attain their goals in recovery and beyond.

Within twelve-step philosophy, the concept of simplicity is often understood as "doing the next right thing." For example, if a young person walks into a twelve-step meeting for the first time and other members suggest they find a sponsor and work the twelve steps, they may feel overwhelmed, especially if they imagine they must interview many people to find the perfect candidate or if they believe all twelve steps must be completed straightaway. However, the recommendation placed before them succinctly outlines the primacy of their needs; and if they choose to acknowledge this solution, they can simply ask someone who possesses firsthand knowledge of the twelve steps to be a sponsor, follow instructions given by their sponsor in regard to working each of the twelve steps, and then make themselves available to sponsor the next newcomer.

Similarly, those new to yoga may feel bewildered when they attempt to fathom the many dimensions of a physical practice, such as numerous styles of poses, variations and modifications for certain postures, specific transitions within established sequences, and special breathing techniques that apply to both moments of action and stillness. However, new or experienced practitioners can simply practice one pose at a time and breathe one breath at a time, and they will be eligible to receive the full benefits of their practice regardless of their personal knowledge or beliefs about yoga.

ACTION AND INACTION, TIME AND SPACE

Although recovery can be characterized by actions one takes to transcend the bondage of addiction in order to move forward in life, without proportionate measures of intelligent inaction—for example, pausing if necessary, resting as needed, or remaining silent when appropriate—continuity and contentment can't be sustained and recovery becomes unbalanced. When those in recovery realize that both action and inaction contribute to the functionality of simplicity, equipoise is revealed to be a fundamental element of this perennial quality.

Imagine if you were to run the entirety of a marathon without managing your pace or replenishing your body with a drink of water. Imagine if you were to remain awake for the next three days without sleeping at night. Imagine if you were to drive a car using the accelerator pedal only and never employing the brakes. Clearly these examples and the decision-making behind them contradict the nature of simplicity since such actions would likely contribute to an overall state of psychological unease, numerous physical complications, and several social hazards.

In addition to the dualism of action and inaction, the interdependence of time and space must be considered to comprehend the full import of simplicity. For example, the next right thing for a person in recovery may be to do today what could have been done yesterday in order to bring about a pleasant tomorrow. Or perhaps nothing new could be done today so that whatever might have been done yesterday can naturally flourish unperturbed by further considerations. Or maybe we must allow something distinct to cease to exist today so that something unknown can be born in its place tomorrow. Clearly these examples underline how the intricacies of a personal time-space continuum and implicit social and global responsibilities correlate with the tenets of simplicity.

LET'S MAKE THIS PERSONAL

Read the questions below. Pause to reflect on your answers. Some responses may be completed with a simple yes or no; others may require further inquiry. Most importantly, recognize the next right thing for you within these scenarios in relation to your overall well-being.

What can you do to simplify your life right now? Can you discard material things within your home that no longer serve a purpose? Can you let go of old ideas within your mind that no longer serve your highest self? Can you sit down to pay a bill, compose a business letter, or forward a personal message to someone who may be waiting to hear from you? Can you make a list of positive qualities and work toward becoming these things? Can you do something to strengthen a particular relationship within your family or circle of friends? Do you need to release a personal daydream or childhood fantasy? Do you need to end an unhealthy relationship or friendship or set a proper boundary with a neighbor or coworker? Is there an action you can take to advance your career? Do you have a medical issue to address or rectify? Can you schedule a personal healing treatment, arrange a recreational activity with like-minded peers, or plan a vacation or similar form of relaxation?

What can you do today for your recovery? Are there amends you owe that can be made? Do you need to write a moral inventory and share it with your sponsor or spiritual advisor? Can you list current personal fears and discuss them with a therapist or trusted friend? Can you attend a twelve-step meeting or similar gathering for those in recovery? Can you help a sober friend by supporting their personal challenges? Are you interested in listening to a recovery-based audio recording, reading a book about recovery or self-development, or viewing a documentary about the biomechanics of addiction and recovery? Can you call an active alcoholic or addict to ask how they are doing and listen with compassion to their response? Can you take a nap, walk in nature, or find a similar respite from your program of action?

What is the next right thing for your spiritual development? Can you deepen your practices of prayer and meditation? Do you feel inspired to study sacred scriptures or similar texts? Are you interested in attending a yoga class? Can you participate in a mindfulness-based workshop? Can you freely offer your time, skills, or resources to anyone in need? Is there someone you can forgive in order to set both of you free? Can you ask another person for forgiveness in relation to something you may have done? Can you address a specific issue in regard to self-forgiveness? Can you visit with your inner child and let them know that you are present and available to support any unfulfilled desires? Can you bring a creative desire from within your soul to fruition? Can you place your hands over your heart and repeat a favorite mantra or affirmation? Can you perform exercises or mindful movements to unify your mind, body, and spirit? Can you find a quiet place to breathe with awareness and cultivate *nirvikalpa*, or inner stillness, so that you can connect to a God or higher power of your own understanding?

CONSEQUENCES OF AVOIDING THE NEXT RIGHT THING

When we avoid simply doing what needs to be done in any area of life, repercussions are commensurate with the degree these activities are necessary or inevitable. For example, if a person with a toothache does not take action when the discomfort is first experienced, an infection may spread; eating or speaking can become difficult; pain can increase; and gum disease or tooth decay may result. If another person chooses not to file a tax return when due, fees and penalties will accrue; a federal audit may be issued; personal wages can be garnished; and access to assets may be restricted. If yet another person does not change the oil within a gas-powered car in a timely manner, this can lead to decrease in fuel economy; increase in harmful atmospheric emissions; certain parts within the mechanism of the engine can become defective; and complete engine failure may be experienced.

When we delay or refuse to simply do the next right thing in recovery for whatever reason—laziness, uncertainty, unwillingness, skepticism, or self-absorption—the resultant procrastinations and postponements water seeds of anxiety, stress, and fear within our consciousness, and our senses and perspective are negatively affected. If we pick and choose when and how to do what needs to be done based on personal whims or favoritism, our comprehension of righteousness erodes. We can't perceive everyday situations with proper objectivity, and relations within all departments of our life become strained. When we are reluctant to perform essential tasks to ensure our sobriety or oppose what is required of us to remain mentally, emotionally, physically, and spiritually fit, issues that are manageable at their inception will seem impossible after repeated deferments. If patterns of avoidance continue, our recovery will likely succumb to all forms of regression. Additionally, when we act out of greed, obsess about outer appearances, or support generational stories and cultural fabrications that do not uplift the collective cognizance of humankind—these manifestations of craving, vanity, and ignorance complicate attempts to determine the next right thing in accordance with our growing understanding of simplicity within recovery.

PRACTICING SIMPLICITY

If we are to surmount all personal defects or shortcomings that are hindering our ability to take the next indicated right action, we will likely need assistance from an omniscient source of power. If we are to set aside personal likes and dislikes and practice impartiality within all endeavors, steadfast guidance from an omnipresent observer will be necessary. If we are to cultivate a mental state of equanimity and undertake all tasks with uniformity of effort, intensity, and enthusiasm, we ought to rely upon the aid of an omnipotent collaborator. And if we are to remain accountable to personal ethical statutes and communal obligations related to all routines for recovery, we have to be willing to accept help from an omnibenevolent source of strength.

Within the yoga tradition, the gayatri mantra is a renowned

ancient Vedic prayer of supplication used by seekers to request and receive divine direction that will enlighten all actions. When such appeals are infused with love and devotion and faith and trust, our finite human intelligence is lifted beyond superficiality toward godly, infinite profundity; our emotionality transcends its lowest natures to reach heavenly heights; our physicality is suffused with limitless reserves of endurance and capability; and our soul is regenerated as the innermost self unifies with its Creator and all of creation.

Below is the gayatri mantra in Sanskrit and a modern interpretation in English. Sing or read these words as a sacred offering to yourself and others. Gather with friends, in person or online, and chant these verses as a unified voice. Use this prayer to overcome whatever is blocking you from doing the next right thing in your life so that you can experience the resplendent and immediate benefits of simplicity.

> *Aum bhur bhuvah suvaha*
> *Tat savitur varenyam*
> *Bhargo devasya dhimahi*
> *Dhiyo yo nah prachodayat*

We meditate on the Divine Light of the Creator of the Universe, whose rays illuminate the entire cosmos. Let's commune with the glory and grace of this Supreme Consciousness so that our mind, body, and spirit become infused with its radiant Reality, and our hearts are protected and guided as we overcome all forms of ignorance to achieve complete enlightenment.

24

Gratitude

Gratitude is the spiritual heart of recovery. Without the energy, power, and multidimensional expression of gratitude, we are unlikely to remain clean and sober. Without the ease and freedom that gratitude affords people who have actively embarked upon a path of discovery in recovery, we can't experience lasting happiness or peace in any area of life. Without gratitude for all the circumstances that have instigated our journey from the darkness and ignorance of active addiction toward the light and intelligence of recovery, and all conditions allowing us to remain and prosper upon this course of continuous unfoldment, we can't maintain conscious contact with our inner light or truth, and we become susceptible to the mortal entrapments of addiction, which include depression, loneliness, boredom, despair, and anger.

Gratitude illumines a path toward unification of the individual, separate self with the universal, absolute substance of all existence. Gratitude can't be perfected through human intelligence or action alone; it is not a personal mental exercise or rational self-discipline, nor is it comprehensible or effectual as an impersonal philosophical concept. True gratitude originates within the heart when the merits of love, compassion, and humility join with an inherent awareness of oneness with all things, appreciation for our particular place within the cosmos, and reverence for divine provisions extended by an immutable and indivisible consciousness that pervades and animates all aspects of reality.

When individual and collective thoughts and prayers of gratitude originate along these lines, they are authentic and whole and prove to be effective and transformational within the lives of those in recovery. When this manner by which gratitude emerges from the heart is truly understood and practiced, its personal benefits, including nonattachment, unselfishness, satisfaction, fearlessness, and exultation, are received with every expression of our thankfulness offered to all people, places, and things that contribute to the unitive nature of life.

CAUSES FOR GRATITUDE

Within the lives of all human beings, infinite causes for gratitude exist. Any person at almost any time anywhere in the world can be thankful when the heart beats, when the lungs expand and contract, when our veins transport blood throughout the body. We can be thankful when we see a wonderland of shapes and colors with our eyes, hear beautiful music with our ears, smell the perfume of flowers with our nose, taste delicious fruits and vegetables with our mouth, feel a gentle breeze on our skin. We can be thankful when the sun is shining, for this phenomenon offers light and warmth; when rain is falling, for this occurrence nourishes the entirety of the earth; when the moon is full, for this spectacle signals the culmination of a cycle that affects our planet and its people at multiple levels, including astronomical, environmental, and emotional.

For those of us who survive the progressive and malevolent disease of active addiction, we can be most grateful for all conditions that have led to recovery and the *marga*, or spiritual path, that has been revealed to us as a result. When we intimately know the depths of despair and degradation while in the throes of various dependences and we can begin life anew in recovery, this is truly a fortunate occurrence. When we struggle in recovery yet forge ahead despite fears of the unknown, relapses, or other setbacks, and we can continue to develop personal routines that reinforce our program of action to establish continuous sobriety, this is nothing short of a miracle. When we suffer from co-occurring mental disorders, emotional irregularities, physical compulsions, and spiritual maladies associated with various addictions yet we can surmount such conditions to achieve lasting states of equanimity and become upstanding citizens within our community, trustworthy workers at our places of employment, exceptional parents to our children, and identifiable examples of recovery to others seeking liberation from the bondage of addiction, these are all causes for genuine gratitude.

DEVELOPING GRATITUDE

When people in recovery learn the true manner by which gratitude is conceived and ascertain its effectiveness as a boundless and essential practice that involves recognition of individual circumstances, awareness of certain privileges, and acknowledgment of spiritual development, special attention can be placed on three areas that sustain recovery at the required levels of the spiritual, interpersonal, and practical. Let's learn more about these categories and get a sense of all the factors that comprise them as instrumental to both the development of gratitude and the enrichment of recovery.

Gratitude for Brahman, or Ultimate Reality

When you say thank you for all that you have discovered and received in recovery, what are you thinking about and which people are you directing your attention toward? Where does your gratitude go when it leaves your heart? Are your thoughts and words of appreciation directed toward God? A higher power of your own understanding? Do you think about Jesus? Buddha? Krishna? Do you visualize divine incarnations, deities, devas, or avatars from your religious or spiritual tradition? Are your words energetic missives sent out into the universe or nature? Do you contemplate Mother Earth when you express gratitude? Do you think about your highest or innermost self when you are thankful? Do you visualize other living beings or loved ones no longer here in human form when you extend gratefulness? Do you consider anything or anyone else when you cultivate the spirituality of gratitude within recovery?

Gratitude for Gurus, or Teachers

Recovery is not an individual effort. A person can hardly achieve sobriety without the guidance of gurus, or teachers, who direct students and seekers from darkness to light. Who has helped you on your path to recovery? Can you be grateful for sponsors or spiritual advisers? Fellow travelers in recovery and like-minded companions? Have you utilized the services of doctors, therapists, social workers? Have yoga teachers or meditation guides offered techniques and practices to bolster your recovery? Can you call to mind mentors, authors, or perhaps sages, saints, and saviors whose teachings have elevated your consciousness, which in turn affected your recovery? Can you regard your parents as teachers who delivered you from ignorance to enlightenment? Can you look on your children as teachers who allow you to learn selflessness, patience, and unconditional love? Can you be grateful for friends or others who have said something that has altered the direction of your life? Can you venerate your breath as an inner teacher? Can you express gratitude to your mind for its ability to collect, categorize, and recall memories? Can you be thankful for your body and its daily teachings about impermanence? Can you appreciate your spirit and its lessons about immutability and everlastingness? Can you recognize your past or present challenges as teaching moments and be grateful for such opportunities to shift your perspective? Is there anyone or anything else you are grateful for in regard to the interpersonal nature of the *guru-chela*, or teacher-disciple, relationship?

Gratitude for Sadhana, or Daily Practice

Without a consistent program of action or daily design for living in recovery, many people who desire continuous sobriety and happiness will unlikely find what they seek. How do you communicate gratitude for personal routines that sustain your recovery each day? Can you be thankful for a code of ethics that allows you to successfully navigate all difficulties? Can you be grateful for certain principles that help you become the best version of yourself one day at a time? Are you thankful for spiritual tools that help you forgive others? Procedures that help you process grief, loss, sadness? Can you be grateful for mottoes, mantras, or mindfulness techniques that eradicate fear, transform anger, remedy depression, or dispel loneliness? Can you be thankful for protocols that guide you through sudden or unexpected changes such as financial matters, relationship issues, health concerns, or career setbacks? Can you be grateful for strategies to amend harms done to others? Systems to become self-disciplined and selfless? Meditations to establish present-moment awareness? Prayers that help you rise above sexual fantasies and subdue sensual yearnings? Are you grateful for tactics that remove unnecessary ruminations and projections from your thoughts, cynicism and gossip from your speech, expectations and attachments from your actions? Can you be grateful for observances that create peace within your heart, which positively affects the integration and health of your mind, body, and spirit? Are you thankful for reliable and respectful ways to love and serve others? How else do you express gratitude each day for the practicality of your program?

25

Contentment

Contentment in recovery is to be comfortable with where we are when we are there. It is to be at ease with being who we are as the truth of our existence is discovered within the reality of any given moment. It is to be okay with how our past has delivered us to the present and how our thoughts, words, and actions in the here and now determine the quality of our future.

Contentment is an active state of repose to be experienced when we are no longer perturbed by the subtleties or complexities of everyday life. It means to no longer harbor regrets for past mistakes nor allow future expectancies or projections to eclipse present obligations. It means to no longer be needful for anything to satisfy selfish or carnal desires nor to become impassioned or obsessed about things that do not support our svadharma, or personal purpose. It is to no longer seek validation or approval from others nor crave any type of recognition or acknowledgment from outer sources. It is to no longer entertain abstract theories that delay the development of self-actualization or collective enlightenment.

Contentment in recovery is experienced when we make peace with all personal and interpersonal transgressions. If we come to believe that human beings simply do what we can with what we have to offer or contribute to the world within any given moment, we will emotionally separate from egotistical or prideful attachments to what is and psychologically disconnect from expectations of what will be. If we neutralize and eliminate attachments and expectations through steadfast and dependable practices, *samskaras*, or habitual mental patterns, which lead to addictions and similar dependent behaviors, can be replaced with positive alternatives as subtle and gross layers of the mind are harmonized. And if we can identify and transform individual hindrances to right thought, speech, and action as we endeavor toward contentment, we will understand how to think with intelligence, speak with kindness, and act with beneficence on behalf of the evolutionary uplifting of all beings everywhere.

Ultimately, contentment in recovery is established when we choose to abide by specific ideals and protocols that allow us to create and maintain an inner sanctum of *ananda*, or bliss, characterized by alertness without anxiety, cognizance without trepidation, and wakefulness without uncertainty.

CULTIVATING CONTENTMENT

Within the Yoga Sutras, a twofold method to develop *santosha*, or contentment, can be found through examination of *abhyasa*, or persistent practice, and *vairagya*, or nonattachment. Let's explore these complementary concepts to see how they affect the mind in relation to addiction and recovery and how they engender the dynamism of contentment. Let's also consider how synchronization of all aspects of the mind—*manas*, or sense-memory; ahamkara, or identity-ego; *chitta*, or storehouse-consciousness; and buddhi, or enlightenment-intellect—enlivens the body and heart, regulates the breath, and awakens our *sakshi*, or inner pure witness, a process that allows us to perceive that the key to contentment is objectivity about oneself.

Abhyasa

Abhyasa describes methodical, devoted personal practices aimed toward the discontinuation of fluctuations within the mind. Repetition of such practices pacifies and eliminates mental triggers, traumas, causes, and conditions that lead to addictive behaviors by aligning the conscious mind with its subconscious and unconscious realms and unifying various waking and dreaming mental states. If our commitment to abhyasa is unwavering and we are diligent with self-regulation, the principal goal of abhyasa— mental tranquility, clarity, and luminescence—will be achieved, and unwholesome *kamas*, or desires, will no longer rouse addictions or similar habit energies from the depths, peripheries, or surface levels of the mind.

Vairagya

Vairagya is renunciation of mental concepts and attitudes that oppose the radiance of our higher nature. It is detachment from *bhoga*, or worldly pleasures that prevent self-realization. It is dispassion for self-centered concerns, material enticements, sensual indulgences, and obsessive entanglements. It means to forsake personal likes and dislikes in favor of principles and observances that benefit all humanity. Vairagya allows us to dissociate from ephemeral cravings and illusory perceptions that perpetuate negative habits and provoke addictive engagements. Vairagya emboldens us to fulfill our *kula-dharma*, or communal purpose, to become *dhiras*, or calm and wise beings untroubled by human emotionality, unaffected by fleeting passions, undisturbed by finite temptations.

There are four stages of vairagya: *yatamana, vyatireka, ekendriya, vasirara*. Let's consider the tenets and practical solutions inherent to these successive phases to see how a person who suffers from addiction can overcome afflictions and find lasting contentment.

Yatamana

This first stage refers to efforts used to restrain ourselves from partaking in unwholesome habits, sensual pleasures, and addictions.

Imagine an alcoholic wants to take a drink. If they can stop thinking and not act upon this habitual impulse, they can choose to focus instead on their breath. They can attempt to find stillness and just breathe. They can close their eyes to minimize distractions and direct all mentation upon their breath. They can cultivate patience and nondiscrimination as they refrain from judging themselves or wishing things were different in this moment. They can practice acceptance as they yield to this situation. They can also deepen their ability to concentrate as they focus solely on their inhale and exhale as their mind unifies with the rhythm of their breath.

Vyatireka

This second stage refers to awareness of how we are emotionally or otherwise attached to certain objects.

In regard to the aforementioned alcoholic, if they quiet their mind through awareness of breath, they can investigate the patterns of their behavior and determine how they have arrived at the moment when they want to drink. They can identify personal stimuli that lead to harmful activities and can transcend these circumstances. They can begin this process by asking: Which feelings precede my desire to drink? Are my cravings mental or physical? Does a specific memory prompt my need for alcohol? Which emotions arise within my mind in anticipation of quenching my thirst? Are there sensations within my body when I think about drinking? Do I have a visceral or palpable urge to obliterate my consciousness or to escape the reality of the present moment?

During this period of self-inquiry, they may conclude that they are not thirsty at all; perhaps they are lonely or sad or angry or anxious. With compassion and nonjudgment, they can honor and embrace unprocessed emotions or feelings and vow to offer attentiveness and reverence to their body. Armed with awareness of what prompts their compulsion to drink, they can now change their responses to loneliness or sadness or anger or anxiety by visualizing new patterns or habits that will generate happiness and satisfaction.

Ekendriya

This third stage refers to attempts to separate our senses from sensations that lead to detrimental habits and destructive patterns.

When the alcoholic in our example acknowledges that old, harmful strategies for dealing with emotions and other triggers are no longer viable, they can use proper discernment to recognize how specific sentiments arise within their mind, heart, and body. They can name their emotions and feelings, accept them as integral to their disposition, and appreciate all parts of themselves without prejudice. They can now learn how their feelings are embodied, and when they become familiar with these somatic effects, they can select and initiate new behaviors or activities to accompany corresponding physiological sensations.

For example, if they realize their chest tightens when they are lonely, they can choose to walk in nature when this symptom shows up. If they realize their shoulders slump forward when they are sad, they can call their sponsor or a trusted friend to talk about their problems when they feel this physical degeneration. If they realize their lower back aches when they are angry, they can take a warm bath when pain arises within this area. If they realize their breathing is labored or their heart rate quickens when they are anxious, they can remove themselves from their surroundings and pray for inner quietude when these sensations occur. As they proceed along these lines, new and positive neural pathways will replace karmic imprints upon their psyche that once led to repetition of habits that did not serve their highest good.

Vasirara

This final stage refers to total dispassion toward stimuli that lead to temptations or addictions.

When our alcoholic observes the previous three stages persistently and wholeheartedly and integrates their results into all areas of their life, they will no longer be predisposed to act upon old, destructive instincts. They will not be enslaved by conditioned behaviors or habitual energies. They will not be besieged by unprocessed emotions or feelings. They will not be enticed by the lure of substances, dependencies, unwholesome activities, or corrosive relationships. They will not be seduced by cultural standards or swayed by societal demands. All aspects of their mind will be quieted and unified, and they will know true happiness and satisfaction. Their thoughts, words, and actions will reflect an inner dimension imbued with independence, gratification, and lucidity. Their senses will be attuned to the dynamics of their body, and they will understand all aspects of their physiology. Their contented presence will reflect the power of an incandescent spirit that can offer refuge to others who seek healing and serenity within their lives.

LET'S MAKE THIS PERSONAL

What is preventing you from experiencing contentment in the present moment? Can you let go of an expectation? An attachment? An old idea that certain conditions must be in place before contentment is possible?

194 *Recovery with Yoga*

Can you recognize a relationship between acceptance and contentment? Surrender and contentment? Open-mindedness and contentment?

How can you bring contentment to others? How can your thoughts positively influence the collective energy of your community? How can your words or actions help all beings everywhere feel satisfaction and ease and freedom?

26

Wholeness

Wholeness in recovery means to be conscious of the many facets of our human constitution and the need for integration and harmony at all levels. It is to preserve mental soundness, emotional sobriety, physical fitness, spiritual acuity. It is to be aware of the psychological and physiological functions of the central and peripheral nervous systems. It is to be mindful of the interplay between the respiratory and circulatory systems and their association with the skeletal and muscular systems. It is to also be familiar with the independent and interdependent functionality of the digestive, endocrine, lymphatic, urinary, reproductive, and excretory systems.

Wholeness in recovery involves maintenance of oral and dental hygiene; care for auditory, visual, and olfactory capacities;

protection of dermatological health. It is regulating natural and supplemental absorption of essential vitamins and minerals. It is properly hydrating the body and its organs. It is keeping the muscles, tendons, and fascia flexible and resilient. It is honoring and managing sexual impulses and other biochemical phenomena that affect the unity of mind, body, and spirit. It is supplying the body with optimal nutrition and adequate rest. It is also properly allocating personal time, attention, and energy in the areas of education and study; work and creativity; recreation and exercise; family and community interests; religious and spiritual observances.

Wholeness in recovery can ultimately be viewed as a methodology to conform with our daily personalized requirements so we remain inwardly and outwardly attentive, empathetic, and energized. We can then intentionally observe and minister to the many facets of our temperament; faithfully endeavor to maintain homeostasis among all aspects of our composition; and earnestly attempt to dissolve divisions between physical, subtle, and causal levels of our humanity so our overall health can be optimized to sustain all stages of recovery.

A YOGIC VIEW OF WHOLENESS

In the Taittiriya Upanishad, a Vedic-era yogic text, five *koshas*, or sheaths, are outlined as a means to apprehend the diversity of our inner and outer lives as individual human beings. When we reconcile such findings with our goal to remain recovered from the hopelessness and aimlessness of active addiction, wholeness is attained through awareness of the properties inherent to each interdependent layer.

Let's analyze the five koshas to see how to synchronize the interpenetration of their respective energy fields—physical, vital, mental, wisdom, bliss—so we can remain free from the bondage of addictions and similar compulsions or ailments. Let's also realize how consideration of the koshas helps us fulfill a collective yogic purpose to become jivanmuktas, or enlightened living beings, who have acquired *jnana*, or experiential wisdom of the true self within all sentient things.

Annamaya Kosha—**Physical**

This first, outermost sheath is composed of physical body energies, which include the cellular and molecular makeup of skin, bones, muscles, organs, nerves, tissues. This is the heaviest and densest layer of our being. It is nourished by *anna*, or edible food, and purified and strengthened by asanas, or yoga poses. When we are cognizant of *annamaya,* the human body can be viewed as our earthly *alaya*, or dwelling, through which the infinitude of the spirit performs right actions within an animate world. When we recognize how our innate spirituality is humanized through sensory and bodily conceptualizations and manifests as active demonstrations of inner and outer harmony and peace, we will intuit our infinite place within the cosmos and dedicate all finite faculties toward reverence for the body and its well-being.

Pranamaya Kosha—**Vital**

This second sheath hovers and radiates beneath annamaya. It is associated with vitality and consists of prana, or life-force energy, that flows through an intricate whole-body system of thousands of nadis, or energetic channels. Within *pranamaya*, the chakras, or wheels of energy along the length of the spine, abide and receive energetic sustenance. Pranamaya is strengthened through pranayama, or breathing techniques and exercises that extend the life force within the entirety of the body. Yogis utilize *bandhas*, or energetic locks, to control the flow of prana; and mudras, or hand gestures, to collect and redirect prana throughout the extremities. Pranamaya can also be invigorated through activities outdoors in nature that allow the rays of the sun to safely penetrate our skin. Additional ways to stimulate pranamaya include subtle-body and homeopathic healing modalities such as acupuncture, reflexology, and *abhyanga*, an Ayurvedic oil massage that focuses on pressing upon *marmas*, or reservoirs of prana, positioned throughout the body.

Manomaya Kosha—**Mental**

This third sheath pulsates and rests below the territories of physical and vital. *Manomaya* is associated with the totality of our mentality. It is where thoughts and emotions are processed, calibrated, and stored. It is where the senses interpret and internalize outer surroundings, relationships, and similar stimuli. It is also where *granthis*, or mental knots, form as the result of unprocessed cognitive complexes, emotional challenges, sentimental entanglements, and narcissistic preferences. Granthis and related cerebral conditions within manomaya can be untangled through use of mantras, or affirmative chants that protect the mind, and then neutralized and rehabilitated through pratyahara, or sensory withdrawal practices, so that reasoning can support the optimization of all internal emotive and sensory analyses.

Vijnanamaya Kosha—**Wisdom**

This fourth sheath lies beneath the physical, vital, and mental layers. It is an access point to intuitive wisdom. It is the repository where intellectual inference is accessible as inner knowing when we become aware of the alliance between matter and spirit. It is where personal morality and willpower merge with universal laws and divine inspiration. *Vijnanamaya* is nurtured through study and application of spiritual truths. For example, yogis who abide by Patanjali's yamas, or moral codes, and niyamas, or self-disciplines, can cultivate sustained states of clarity along with heightened levels of creativity and arrange their lives according to inner guidance received through enhanced instinctual capabilities. *Dhyana*, or meditation, is also a helpful means to comprehend the dimensions of vijnanamaya since such an inwardly directed venture allows practitioners to access prajna, or deep insight, then make good use of direction sourced from inner realms of higher intelligence.

Anandamaya Kosha—**Bliss**

This final, fifth sheath resides beyond the others yet substantiates the properties and potencies available within each layer of the self. *Anandamaya* is the bliss sheath. It is our inmost source of unbridled joy and boundless peace. It is the thin partition that veils the unmistakable luster at the center of our being. Anandamaya is realized through soul-searching inquiries and disciplines that help us identify the truth of our relationship with the atman, or innermost self, in relation to Brahman, or our highest self or God within. *Kirtan*—a yogic devotional practice of chanting the names of God—is a means to enter into ecstatic states of blessedness and reverie so we can touch the reality and splendor of anandamaya. Seva, or selfless service, is an additional method to fortify anandamaya since thoughts, words, and actions can be offered as expressions of unconditional love from the bliss within our hearts to all humankind.

LET'S MAKE THIS PERSONAL

Do you associate with any of these layers of self more than the others? For example, do you find yourself fixated on your physical appearance? Can you recognize if your breath is shallow when you are anxious or if you hold your breath when you are fearful? Do you spend too much time thinking about past emotional experiences? Do you remain open-minded in regard to learning or studying various topics of interest? Do you arrange your schedule to prioritize spiritual practices?

How can you best allocate your time, energy, and attention evenly among the five layers of self in order to achieve wholeness in recovery?

27

Community

Within a community of people in recovery, an alcoholic or addict entrapped in the prison of individualism can awaken to find companionship among a collective of like-minded seekers who have achieved liberation from the confinements of behavioral and chemical dependences. Within this type of regenerative community, the ego can't wreak havoc in the minds of sober people since opportunities to think of others abound when time is spent amid kindred spirits. When such communities are populated with people who desire complete healing and transformation, practical solutions to personal issues that impede lasting recovery can be sourced in collaboration with others who are also seeking support for the quality and duration of their sobriety.

Recovery communities thrive when members dedicate time and energy to the development and integration of wholesome communal ideals in their lives and adhere to the daily maintenance such a lifestyle necessitates. Concurrently, when members of a recovery community independently practice principles that substantiate their shared program of action, the moral credibility of the group as a whole is upheld; its reputation for efficacy remains positive; and nonmembers and other sufferers find inspiration and wellness alongside its resident exemplars.

Through the spirit of a recovery community, individual goals and dreams are realized when we recognize that assistance is a matter of proximity, and all members within the group hold keys to locks that hinder particular achievements of personal aspirations. When we identify and entrust certain mentors or role models to guide us toward accomplishments we can't solely bring to fruition, private challenges are overcome as our individual consciousness is suffused with the intelligence of a collective consciousness that protects its contributors from egoism, separateness, and mediocrity. Similarly, inner struggles and outer battles can be resolved when solutions are worked out in the company of those who have overcome comparable predicaments and the details of their journey are articulated as experiential wisdom gleaned from openhearted revelations acquired through personal reflection and assimilation.

EVERY PERSON MATTERS IN A RECOVERY COMMUNITY

Without the symbiotic relationships that develop between participants in a recovery community, the group can't thrive. If members are unwilling to receive and extend aid to all who seek guidance throughout the various stages of addiction and recovery, personal sobriety is jeopardized without the hallmarks of a robust recovery community of identification, sympathy, and selflessness. If a recovery community doesn't have a sense of unity, the group will unlikely retain its singleness of purpose. It may splinter into varying factions, as members lose continuous sobriety and newcomers and others who meet inclusionary requirements are deprived of a sanctuary where reversal of unhealthy degenerative conditions is possible.

Addiction has no preferences for the people it attacks. It does not care about our race, creed, caste, or color. It does not care about our age or gender. It does not care if we are educated or not, wealthy or not, healthy or not. It does not care which languages we speak. It does not care about our spiritual or secular affiliations. It does not care if we have families or friends. It also does not care which of its substances or behaviors ultimately confounds, devastates, defeats, or kills us.

If those in a recovery community are to withstand mental affronts, emotional woundings, physical harms, and spiritual barriers positioned before us each day by the minions of addiction, there can't be superficial divisions among members. If addiction does not discriminate against its prey, people in recovery must recognize and use this to their advantage. Simply, if addiction *targets* everyone, recovery communities must *welcome* everyone and honor all contributions of each member.

Recovery communities typically comprise those who are familiar with the battleground of addiction. When our lives are at risk, we need the closeness of others who know the gravity of our shared malady. We need advice from those who have been where we have been. We need the wisdom of people who have fought and won wars against dependencies and similar disorders and diseases. We need to regularly hear about hard-earned experiences so that we do not endure unnecessary pain or misery. We need members who know how to remain strong so that others can rely on them in times of trouble. We need elders who can teach newcomers that outer differences or discriminative factors must never divide us. We need those who relapse to remind us that the forces of addiction are still active in the world. We need those who are tranquil to teach us how to remain levelheaded in all situations. We need those who are pragmatic to tell us how to take right action no matter the cost. We need all members to know how to give and receive constructive feedback. We need people who can speak lovingly so that when we share stories and suggestions, our tone is authentic and encouraging. We need people who can listen with compassion so that whatever weighs heavy on the minds and hearts of our brethren can be unburdened. We need stalwarts to support the community and its ideals despite what may arise in relation to the inner and outer workings of the group. We need caretakers to minister to members who are weak, vulnerable, lonely, or sick. We need all contributors to be a benevolent presence in the face of hatred or anger or judgment and offer kindness and tolerance and acceptance as antidotes. We need helpers to hold our hand when we are scared; friends to encourage us with kind words, a smile, or hug when we are lost or confused; companions to illuminate the space around us when we see nothing but darkness; and allies to celebrate all our victories with us.

A YOGIC PERSPECTIVE ON
COMMUNITY-BUILDING

Within the yoga tradition, the term *kula* denotes a "family" or "community." It is a group within which individuals find a sense of belonging alongside others who have similar aspirations. In a kula, shared values are upheld as certain universal guidelines are observed by all participants. When members of a kula gather, the atmosphere is welcoming, inclusive, and inspiring; it is a safe and peaceful environment, infused with the energy of solidarity or oneness, whereby personal and interpersonal harmonious relations are created and sustained.

Kulas remain active and influential when members meet frequently to develop personal and interpersonal qualities that strengthen the integrity and longevity of the group. Kulas stay intact and continue to be beneficial when autonomous and egalitarian frameworks provide solid structures by which members govern themselves through the power and unanimity of a collective voice. Kulas become sacred spaces when adherents offer equal amounts of kindliness and the same degrees of affection and understanding to all participants. Additionally, if kulas synthesize structural components of *satsangs*, or spiritual communities—such as meditations, explorations of truth, study of scriptures or relevant texts, and open forums for discussions—with the functionality of their essential tenets and observances, constructive societies will be founded and attendees can experience personal growth and spiritual development.

If those who wish to establish sustainable recovery communities familiarize themselves with the philosophies and practices inherent in kulas and satsangs and implement pertinent discoveries alongside the general requirements for their respective groups, extraordinary congregations can be formed and all members will benefit. If recovery remains the foremost purpose for all gatherings, revitalization of the mind, body, and spirit for each member is inevitable. And if the qualities of *maitri*, or friendliness; karuna, or compassion; *mudita*, or joy; and upeksha, or impartiality, are cultivated within the hearts of all members, their thoughts, words, and actions will be suffused with perennial wisdom.

A PRACTICE FOR COMMUNITY-BUILDING

Yoga Sutra 1.33 states:

Maitri karuna mudita upeksanam sukha duhka punya visayanam bhavanatah citta prasadanam

This Sanskrit aphorism can be translated as follows: "When we cultivate an attitude of friendliness toward those who are happy, compassion toward those who are unhappy, joy for those who are virtuous, and impartiality for those who are nonvirtuous, the mind remains undisturbed and calm."

Meditation on the illimitable qualities and equable attitudes within this sutra can provide members of any recovery community opportunities to contemplate and understand how to develop mutual trust and respect; form unique and lasting friendships; increase *titiksa*, or the will and power to endure; and create distinctive havens for personal and collaborative wellness and renewal.

Below is a guided meditation to assist those who desire to be an integral part of a recovery community. Read these lines slowly and deliberately. Breathe with awareness as you consider the meaning of each statement. Internalize these concepts so they can inform all your personal interactions and relationships. Envision how to incorporate these ideas into the ethos of your recovery community.

May all beings be happy, and may all beings be able to cultivate and feel happiness always.

May all beings be free from unnecessary suffering, and may all beings be able to transmute all pains and sorrows in order to learn and grow from such experiences.

May all beings be joyful, and may all beings be able to generate joy for themselves and others at any time.

May all beings be free from any sense of separation, and may all beings be able to accept people, places, and things as they are in the present moment.

28

Service

Service is the golden thread that unifies all facets of recovery. It stitches together our individual characteristics with universal principles so we may become unselfish and thus useful in every situation within each moment of our lives. Service hems together a recovered mind, regenerated body, and renewed spirit so we can fulfill a collective purpose to truly understand and love all beings. When acts of service originate from the purity of the heart and indomitability of the soul, they are initiated with human will and power yet interwoven and perfected by divine assistance, as God never forsakes the selfless or tenderhearted or faithful.

Being of service is the secret to sobriety. It frees us from egotistical prisons of self-centeredness. It lifts us above traps of self-adoration and morasses of self-absorption and self-involvement.

It allows us to circumvent the toxicity of narcissism so long as we continue to place preferential attention upon the welfare of others rather than oneself.

When an objective to serve others remains a preeminent part of our program of action, individual desires to drink alcohol, use drugs, or engage in similar behaviors diminish; private schemes that threaten the well-being of our families and communities dissolve; and unwholesome plans that may separate us from the safety and security of conscious awareness of our Creator disappear. When our thought forms are predominated by inquests of how to serve those in need, both the quality and extent of our recovery are strengthened since higher realms of mental and spiritual clarity are activated by the intentionality of altruism.

Recovery without service is mechanical, robotic. Without consistent consideration for the daily necessities of others, recovery becomes stale, stagnant. If the essential requirements of those we feel impelled to serve are not prioritized before personal wants or desires, progression of recovery and expansion of its dynamism are improbable until we capitalize on mutually beneficial opportunities for spiritual growth and development. For instance, if we offer nourishment to a person who is hungry, our capacities for selflessness, charitableness, and generosity deepen while the recipient of our concerns and contributions feels acknowledged, accepted, and loved. If we give time and energy to a person who feels lonesome or depressed, our abilities to offer consolation and encouragement improve while the beneficiary of our companionship and sympathy feels heartened and hopeful. If we remain calm and peaceful when confronted by a person who is angry or argumentative, our inclinations to be understanding and patient in all situations increase while mental and emotional insecurities or hostilities de-escalate and neutralize within the mind and heart of the individual in our presence.

Service in recovery ought never to be considered a hindrance to our schedule, nor should we feel that our vitality will be depleted when we help others. Rather, each thought, word, or deed expended in the name of service can be perceived as an investment to maintain our sanity and mature our sobriety. If service seems burdensome to a person in recovery, an immediate attitude adjustment is required until service is understood as a sacred, human obligation to follow what is universally identified as the Golden Rule—to do unto others as we would have done unto us.

Service in recovery ought to be carried out freely and cheerfully without expectation of reward, recognition, or remuneration. We should take action calmly, with humility and anonymity, and try to be legitimately helpful to those in need within the reality of the present moment. We should remain unattached to our works and indifferent toward any fruits of our labor. We should also allow people to be of service to us during our times of need and accept all relevant offerings with grace and gratitude, lest we deprive others opportunities to internalize the benefits of selflessness and helpfulness.

If we ignore requests to be of service or refuse to acknowledge the hardships of those around us or give precedence to personal whims and obsessions rather than the welfare of communal relations, a unique and haunting type of regret reserved for the self-obsessed plagues the mind, and ruminations inspired by indecisiveness and guilt may be experienced. If we offer service begrudgingly or maliciously, a singular form of remorse permeates the subtle body, and physical pains, in addition to similar internal maladies, may be incurred. If we are unwilling to master the balance of hospitality and service within any area of our lives, a shroud forged by the pairing of vanity and idleness darkens the radiance of the spirit, and our proclivity and aptitude to remain in recovery may contract, for without awareness of mutuality with others in recovery and heartfelt attempts to symbiotically offer and receive healing and happiness, we can't realize or retain personal homeostasis.

Service normalizes the particulars of personal sobriety by opening the aperture of the mind, which allows us to recognize the collectivity of human experience. Service civilizes and synchronizes our layers of consciousness as the pluralistic plights of humankind are considered, instead of self-pitying analyses or similar egotistic indulgences. Service spiritualizes the firmament of our recovery by softening and enlarging the dimensions of the human heart so we can sense all animate hearts are creatively, energetically, and divinely conjoined.

SERVICE AS SPIRITUAL PRACTICE

Yogic philosophy extols the virtues of seva, or selfless service, as a means to extend kindhearted care to others while simultaneously cultivating the spiritual dimension of our lives. Through this qualitative act of giving love, energy, time, and other wholesome assets from the depths of the heart—rather than quantitatively offering things from the edifices of ego, reputation, or superiority—our *pratyaksa*, or perception, is clarified and uplifted so we can view all beings as manifestations of an absolute source that sustains all forms of life.

When such a *sahaja prajna*, or innate insight of oneness, is awakened within the mind, love and devotion for God—or Light, or truth, or Christ consciousness, or buddha-nature, or whichever designation one chooses to signify the centermost entity of existence—becomes our motivation to forever comfort others as we will intuitively know that this unparalleled practice, which can be categorized as a form of Karma Yoga, honors the highest self within all beings, ourselves included.

Without a visionary perspective of the divine in others, the primary personal benefits of seva—peacefulness and purposefulness—can't be ascertained or acquired. Unless we are willing to selflessly offer beneficent thoughts, words, and actions to our conception of God indwelling within all beings, true happiness or lasting joy can't be attained. And until the limited notion of selfhood is abolished from our consciousness and we come to believe all humans exist interdependently and our hearts are divinely united, God-realization is unlikely to be possible.

When we identify the glory of God within all peoples and practice seva discreetly and consistently, *adambhitvam*, or pridelessness, is the spiritual gift bestowed upon us. Possession of this honorable trait allows for *parashakti*, or supreme creative power, to circulate unobstructed throughout the mind and body. This animating force enthuses us on the mortal and material planes of existence to accomplish individual ventures within specific vocations distinctly aligned with our prakriti, or comportment. It inspires and energizes us to fulfill our collective spiritual destiny to love and serve all living things.

When we bear in mind that all beings are incarnations of one Blessed Presence, and we act favorably on behalf of the welfare of all creatures, our behavior will likely be positive and beget like results. Jnana, or wisdom of the self as inseparable from the divine, will be the reward. When we choose not to envision a Lord of Love within the heart of every living thing and act unfavorably or in opposition to this spiritual truth, we will likely draw negative circumstances into our lives that reflect and reinforce our disbelief and disobedience; *moha*, or lack of understanding and confusion about the true nature of the relationship between the self and others and the divine, will then dictate an undesirable direction for our lives. Therefore, the implacability of our karma, which can be interpreted as an impressionable and causal type of fate based on the nature of our actions, is undeniably affected by seva.

A PRAYER FOR SERVICE

The following prayer can be recited each morning to direct our thoughts, words, and actions toward how we can best serve others. Use this prayer to complement your existing spiritual practice. Share it with friends in recovery. Be willing to listen for the answers that will come if these words are spoken in earnest from the heart. And be willing to act on any spiritual or intuitive direction that you receive.

God, please allow me the willingness, eagerness, presence, patience, and passion to know when, where, and how to be of service in every situation I am in today if it be Thy will.

29

Authenticity

When we get clean or sober and find recovery, we have an opportunity to know and establish a relationship with our authentic self. This can be a worrisome or frightening consideration for former alcoholics and addicts, since many of us have spent a lot of time deliberately avoiding self-identification through periodic or regular use and abuse of certain mood-altering substances and self-destructive behaviors. However, unless we endeavor throughout recovery to understand and accept our authentic self and find union with this inner source of wisdom, we will be unlikely to experience a total transformation to become the people we are here to be and live the life we are here to live.

When we are stuck in active addiction, a cloak of superficiality separates us from our actual interior life, and we are incapable of realistically processing the multidimensionality and interdependence of our feelings, emotions, memories, perceptions, and experiences. Similarly, when addiction takes possession of our conscience, we can't fathom the veracity of our exterior life, appropriately interact within personal relationships, or effectively participate in worldly matters. Therefore, we need to cleanse the cognitive, causal remnants of addiction from our consciousness with various holistic, curative modalities including psychological treatment, emotional healing, behavioral therapy, and spiritual practices, or both our inner and outer life in recovery will suffer since we will not be able to fully acquaint ourselves with the genuine intelligence of our authentic self, and consequently, our thoughts, words, and actions will not be aligned with its virtuous guidance.

THE PRESENCE OF OUR AUTHENTIC SELF

The authentic self is integral to our innate disposition and forever dwells within every human being. In infanthood, it manifests as spontaneous and joyous smiling. In childhood, it expresses as instinctive curiosity and creativity. In adolescence, it exhibits as intuition to seek clarity about the nature of humanity and the general meaning of life. In adulthood, it inspires us to speak and act on behalf of truth, equality, and peace and to cultivate a spiritual relationship with a higher power of our own understanding.

In active addiction, the authentic self is the internal voice that encourages us to steadfastly endure the struggles and consequences that come from our unwholesome behaviors. It is the subtle energy that lets us know we have more to offer the world than the words and actions stemming from the stupors of our disease. It is the intrinsic knowingness that convinces us we possess adequate strength to overcome our problems and, when conditions are right, we will lift ourselves above our current circumstances.

In recovery, the authentic self is the entity that identifies what is best for us on our continuous journey toward wellness and informs and instructs us accordingly. It is the motivating influence that helps us gradually refine our personality so we can generate personal happiness and contentment and offer the fruits of these universal qualities to others. It is the gentle provocation that rouses us to regularly participate in meaningful experiences in order to find ingenious growth and spiritual development.

The authentic self is our unparalleled true nature. It continuously seeks our highest good as it intrinsically works out details and designs to bring about fulfillment of our purpose within this lifetime. Whether we choose to call the authentic self our inner essence, soul, spirit, source, or some other name, we can trust that it will never abandon us, lead us awry, or fail to bring us to our rightful place within the world in perfect time and space so long as we remain willing to hear, integrate, and follow it within all areas of our lives.

BECOMING AUTHENTIC

Within the yoga tradition, the word *bhava* can be interpreted as "becoming." It means to return to ourselves in the present moment in order to determine our *svabhava*, or individual sense of identity and purpose. Yogis commence this process through Nada Yoga, or deep inner listening; Dhyana Yoga, or meditation and coincident assimilation; and Karma Yoga, or implementation and embodiment of right action.

When we investigate the nature of our interiority utilizing these yogas and their comprehensive practices, we can procure an awareness of our authentic self or the immanent witness within, and *visarga*, or a sending forth and release of that which comes from inner revelations, is the result. These emanations then develop into *spanda*, or pulsations of creative spiritual energies, which underlie and sustain all cosmic movement, as our authentic self becomes synchronized with the ritam, or rhythm of the cosmos. *Anubhava*, or a sublime sense of personal peace and stillness, is the culmination of these inner workings as we outwardly become the singular person we are here to be.

Let's examine the aforementioned yogas to learn how to achieve union with our authentic self in order to fully realize the existence we are here to personify.

Nada Yoga

The Sanskrit word *nada* can be defined as "sound." To perceive messages from our authentic self, we must foster receptivity to hear both inner sounds and inner silences. We must learn to discern which of these sounds and silences are pleasant and unpleasant, natural and unnatural, necessary and unnecessary. We must also be willing to perfect our ability to listen only to what is intoned by the authentic self, while we may likely need to disregard the disquieting whispers of the ego, disparagements voiced by addiction, clamors of external worldly noise, and other such resonances that tend to drown out *vak*, or audible and inaudible sounds and vibrations, from our true nature.

Dhyana Yoga

The Sanskrit term *dhyana* is typically defined as "meditation." However, it can also be broken down to the root words *dhi*, which can be interpreted as "to perceive or think or reflect," and *yana*, which can be defined as "a path or course or journey." Additionally, the root word for *yoga* is *yuj*, which means "to yoke or unite." Therefore, Dhyana Yoga can be viewed as an active process by which we mentally contemplate and consciously internalize a specific subject or points of focus to achieve a state of clarity and coherency by which we unify and attain oneness with our authentic self.

Karma Yoga

The Sanskrit word *karma* means "action." To achieve freedom and peace through Karma Yoga, we must first look within ourselves to determine how personal suffering and selfishness manifest and remove the impetuses and causes of these hindrances so we can offer what originates within our heart to others without attachment to the results of our actions. When the heart is purified in this way, we can properly ascertain what our authentic self wants us to do and be and give full awareness and dedication to the fulfillment of its wishes and plans for our life span.

PRACTICING AUTHENTICITY

The following threefold practice integrates contemplative features from Nada, Dhyana, and Karma Yoga so practitioners can embark on an inner journey to become *sthitaprajnas*, a yogic term that delineates those who have achieved a calm and contented state of existence or being with the mind fixed firmly on the wisdom of the innermost self.

Allow the effects of this practice to unfold naturally. Be patient as you move through all dimensions of these yogas, some of which may seem independent and linear, while others may feel interdependent and circular. Be accepting of your insights. Be openhearted toward emotions that may manifest. Be considerate if you encounter inner darkness. Be humble if you receive inner illumination. Allow your breath and heart to support you. Keep a notebook and pen nearby to record your reflections. Last, remain open-minded and willing to explore the entirety of your interior life—memories, feelings, attachments, expectations, dreams, and more—and the reward will be conscious contact with your authentic self.

Begin in a quiet, safe location. Assume a comfortable position, perhaps seated or supine. Ask yourself the following questions: "Who am I to be today?" "What am I to do today?" "Who am I to become in this lifetime?" Close your eyes.

Listen as answers to these questions arise from a place of deep inner knowing. Listen for sounds and silences. Listen for energies, memories, fantasies, divine whispers, longings of the heart. Listen for words. Listen for feelings. Listen for recollections from your inner child. Listen for wisdom from your ancestors. Listen for questions from your descendants. Listen for secrets from angels. Listen for the sacred syllables of *Aum* or *Om*. Listen for the voice of God.

Meditate on what has arisen within your mind and heart. Meditate on specific nouns, verbs, principles, silences. Meditate on imaginary and realistic dialogues. Meditate on musical or melodic messages. Meditate on images, ideas, forms, colors, visions, vibrations. Meditate on scenes from your past. Meditate on projections of your future. Meditate on the quality of your breath. Meditate on the rhythm of your heartbeat. Meditate on energetic currents along your spine. Meditate on tingling sensations within your inner and outer body. Meditate on all these things in the reality of now.

Bring awareness to your physical body. Become aware of the dexterity of your hands and the strength of your arms. Become aware of the stability of your feet and the sturdiness of your legs. Become aware of the shape and size of your torso and how it contains and protects your internal organs. Become aware of your sense organs and your abilities to see, hear, smell, taste, and touch. Reach your hands and arms upward—feel the air above you. Reach your feet and legs outward—feel the space around you. Touch and bless the earth below you—feel the solidity and sanctuary of our planet. Take a deep inhale—draw all things from the outer realms of existence into your body. Exhale—send forth all inner revelations as contributions to uplift humanity and the entire cosmos throughout time and space.

To finalize your practice, recite the mantra *Om bhavam namah*, which can be translated as "I am one with my authentic self." This mantra affirms the limitless potentiality and perfection of our inmost being and solidifies our awareness of oneness with all of existence.

30

Vigilance

Vigilance in recovery does mean to be on guard. However, it is not to be on guard out of fear or lack of knowledge. If we didn't already know our enemies or how they attacked, there would likely be cause for fear. But we do know our enemies are alcohol, drugs, and other forms of addiction or disease. We know they attack through cravings, wrong thinking, manipulation of our memories and feelings, and the other methods we've explored throughout this book.

Vigilance in recovery is to be on guard so we never again need to meet, battle, or be defeated by our enemies. It is keeping addictions and negative behaviors in the past by fully inhabiting the present moment. It is creating a future of fearlessness through the practice of principles that lift us above our enemies and their attempts to hinder recovery.

Vigilance is comprehensive, natural, and relevant to all areas of life. It is something all people practice when safety or health are threatened. For example, when intense weather approaches a particular city, its townspeople turn their attention to media outlets, watch and listen to weather reports, acquire information about the storm, and learn to overcome the challenges that extreme weather brings. Or if a group of people are recent cancer survivors and need to be tested twice a year to determine they remain without malignant cancer cells, they will visit the doctor or laboratory, verify their remission status, and follow medical orders to keep cancer-free.

Vigilance is something practiced in all areas of our lives so we can survive. We practice vigilance in recovery so we can both survive and thrive. We practice vigilance in recovery so that judgment and dread will not be able to commandeer our thoughts or actions. We practice vigilance in recovery so that dignity will underlie our decision-making processes and courage will determine the quality of our lives. We practice vigilance in recovery to cultivate right knowledge; to know where we stand emotionally, mentally, physically, and spiritually; to recognize what we are here to do and embody who we are here to be. We practice vigilance in recovery to be able to see oncoming problems and respond proactively and positively rather than react passively and negatively.

Vigilance preserves and protects the treasure of lasting recovery. It sharpens and exemplifies the principles on which we stand. It makes recovery practical and possible rather than theoretical and impossible. It allows those who overcome addiction and disease to humanize recovery. It is how we bear witness to others who struggle with addiction or similar problems, how we show up in the world as ambassadors for healing and transformation, how we transmit hope and the promise of sovereignty to those who desire these things. Imagine if a young person is seeking sobriety and encounters people in recovery who are angry, fearful, and miserable. It is unlikely this person will be attracted to recovery based on what they have witnessed. However, if this person encounters people in recovery who practice vigilance, they will likely meet living examples of conscious awareness, compassion, and contentment. And it is likely they will want to learn more about recovery from people who follow a positive, practical, and principled path.

Lack of vigilance is a primary reason those who struggle with addiction and other forms of disease can't maintain sobriety or abstinence and achieve lasting recovery. Without vigilance, we are defenseless against multiple enemies and their attacks upon our emotional, mental, physical, and spiritual states of being. Without vigilance as an operational part of our day, personal and collective wholeness, happiness, and peace deteriorate. Without vigilance as an active part of our recovery regimen, opportunities for self-sabotage multiply and the foundation of our sobriety can't withstand confrontation or uncertainty. If vigilance does not support all aspects of recovery, sloth manifests in its place; dedication to personal sanity wavers; and chaos ensues in our lives as we forget what we know to be true, falter and succumb to old lures and regretful behaviors, and lose our sense of honor and humanity.

VIGILANCE AT ALL TIMES

In my early sobriety, I overheard the following story about vigilance. Let this serve as a practical demonstration of how vigilance upholds the integrity of recovery for those who choose to honor this principle.

A sober woman sat alone in the first-class section of an airplane. The flight attendant offered her a complimentary alcoholic beverage. The sober woman looked around. She realized that nobody would know if she accepted the drink. She realized that nobody from her hometown or recovery support group would know if she relapsed. She began to romanticize the notion that it would be fun and glamorous to have a cocktail on the plane, in secret, and never tell anyone about it.

Then she recalled the misery and torment of her old drinking life compared to the joy and serenity of her new life in recovery. And she graciously thanked the flight attendant for the offer and requested a cup of water instead.

VIGILANCE AND INNER STRENGTH

Vigilance is strengthened when dedication and concentration are consistently applied to spiritual disciplines and intentional secular activities. It is deepened and ripened through persistence and progression. It is reinforced when enthusiasm and reverence are leveraged to advance us upon a path of personal development. It is fostered when we are well-informed in regard to our personal states of being.

There are many ways to cultivate vigilance. Books, teachers, and various spiritual and secular traditions can provide information on this topic. However, external sources of inspiration rarely offer more than knowledge. When we draw on internal resources of power, we access an infinite wellspring of wisdom that can overcome addiction and safeguard recovery.

Within the yogic tradition, there is a source of inner strength known as *tapas*. The Sanskrit root *tap* means "to burn or illuminate with the heat of transformation." Tapas can be defined as the disciplined use of an inner resource of energy that rids impurities from the mind, body, and spirit. Tapas is an inherent force that drives us toward achieving a goal. It is a power that propels us forward. It is conscious, sustained effort. It is fuel that gets us where we need to be upon our journey through life.

Tapas motivates us to do the right thing when we feel torn, tired, or weak. It is how we apply dedication to recovery. It is likely the last line of defense if we entertain old, negative thoughts that may lead to addictive behavior. Tapas has the power to render temptations ineffective, defend recovery against lapses of judgment, conquer stimuli that elicit wrong perceptions, and replace negative thoughts with right actions.

Tapas allows us to attain the fruits of recovery—freedom, peace, joy, calm, friendship, and more. It allows us to rise above smallness or mediocrity to be our best self. It helps us to trust the progression of recovery so we can use our experiences to help others. It gives us an understanding of the framework of recovery so we can create and maintain a life of meaning and purpose. It helps establish our recovery as genuine and embodied rather than theoretical and transient.

Tapas is cultivated through spiritual alchemy. When we learn to think, speak, and act in ways that incinerate thoughts, words, and deeds that no longer serve our well-being, the limitless power of tapas impels us to become the person God or our higher power would have us be in any given moment. For example, instead of rehashing old stories or excuses within the mind, we can repeat a positive affirmation or mantra. Instead of broadcasting the faults of others, we can keep silent and focus on transforming our own shortcomings. Instead of being lethargic and lamenting the state of the world, we can pick up litter within our neighborhood, join a coalition to end human slavery, feed those who are hungry, or take similar actions to contribute to the welfare of all people everywhere.

Tapas is not an esoteric concept; it is a cosmic law. Heat and fire transform things. When gold is sourced from the earth, it is burned so that impurities can be removed from the precious metal. When we want to prepare food so that it is edible, we place it inside an oven or over a fire. When we want to smell the fragrance hidden within a stick of incense, we use a match or lighter.

When tapas is rightly kindled, vigilance becomes the primary shield protecting the totality of our recovery. We will know this to be true as the power of choice becomes ours and inner and outer changes transpire. We will remain open-minded and teachable. Limiting beliefs will dissipate. Contrary thoughts and actions will lead toward enlightenment. Private anguish will no longer plague our consciousness, and underlying conditions beneath personal compulsions will be healed.

When the forces of vigilance and tapas remain strong and both are practiced sincerely and consistently, we will blaze through challenges and similar circumstances in recovery with integrity and grace as we maintain our soundness of mind. Harmful behaviors will be replaced by beneficial actions as we discover and water seeds of growth and development within all our experiences. We will learn to love ourselves and become capable of loving and serving all beings as we move forward in recovery rather than backward toward addiction. We will confront and eradicate things in our lives that threaten happiness, joy, peace, and calm as we deepen our commitment to upholding personal morality, which will allow our conscience to remain clear.

NOURISHING OUR
INNER STRENGTH

The following suggestions nourish, maintain, and stoke the fire of tapas so that we can remain vigilant and thrive in recovery. Choose a few disciplines from the list below that interest you. Choose a time each day to practice these activities in a manner that suits your personal tastes or traditions. Commit to a plan of action. Do your chosen activities for a specific number of consecutive days. Notice if there are any changes in how you feel about recovery and life. Write down relevant observations and discuss your experiences with a friend. Consider incorporating some of these activities into your daily routine.

Prayer

Meditation

Journaling

Reading spiritual or inspiring literature

Walking in nature

Practicing yoga

Pranayama, or conscious breathing exercises

Playing a musical instrument

Making a gratitude list

Caring for a garden

Putting a puzzle together

Painting or another creative endeavor

Attending a twelve-step meeting or similar gathering with
like-minded peers in recovery

LET'S MAKE THIS PERSONAL

Read and answer the following questions. Internalize your
reactions. Recognize the relevance of vigilance in relation to
your recovery. Recognize how tapas can bolster vigilance within
your life. Recognize where a positive new thought or wholesome
contrary action can be substituted for a negative old idea or
unwholesome conditioned behavior. Call a friend in recovery to
discuss your answers.

Where in your recovery and life can vigilance be helpful? Can
you realize when your thoughts may be wrong? Are you willing
to examine your perspective when you are rigid? Can you admit
when you need help? Are you willing to do whatever is necessary
to save yourself and your sobriety? Can you do the right thing
when nobody is looking? Are you willing to do anything to
maintain the integrity of your recovery? Can you use the tools
you have learned in recovery within all areas of your life?

What does your recovery mean to you? How can you be on
guard against things that attack the quality of your recovery?
What can you do to sharpen your awareness and resilience? How
can you enrich and fortify your recovery? Is there disharmony
between your thoughts, speech, and actions? Which of your old
behaviors or ideas need to be transmuted?

Is there something you need to get past, move through, or
extend beyond? What can you do to shift your life toward something new or better? How can you stoke an inner fire to purify

your perception? How can you light the inner lamp of awareness within your heart? How can you use tapas to forge a new path toward clearer or deeper insight? What stokes the flames of wisdom within your recovery? How do you share the radiance of your recovery with others?

CONCLUSION

The principles and concepts in this book have the potential and power to help you navigate your path of recovery. The practices and self-reflective questions make it possible for you to discover the causes and conditions of your addictive behaviors and find suitable solutions for your current challenges. The exercises and observances provide opportunities to integrate their value into each area of life so that true happiness, freedom, harmony, and peace can be realized.

As the result of your work with the suggestions in this book, your understanding of your mind, body, and spirit will be heightened. Your heart will be more open, compassionate, and forgiving. Your thoughts will be more aligned with your speech and actions. You will be more aware of how to live your life fully and deeply in the present moment. And your recovery will be more embodied and dynamic.

Moving forward, consider how you can continue to develop your recovery or yoga practice. Will you reread this book or similar titles? Listen to recordings and watch videos about yogic philosophy, spirituality, or mindfulness? Attend workshops or trainings to further your studies? Go to twelve-step meetings or similar gatherings in your community or online? Establish and maintain a regular yoga, meditation, prayer, or mantra practice at home or in a studio? Share your experience, strength, and hope with those in need?

RECOVERY AND YOGA ARE BOUNDLESS

Perfection or completion are never the goals within the complementary disciplines of recovery and yoga. In recovery, we simply do our best one day at a time. In yoga, we take one breath at a time, recite one mantra at a time, and do one pose at a time.

Recovery and yoga both provide unlimited opportunities to continue to cultivate personal talents and skills, become more conscious of our unique place in the world, and acquire spiritual tools to solve personal and interpersonal dilemmas. When these practices are developed in the present moment, our realizations remain fresh, creative, and practical. When our efforts remain steady and our perception is allowed to mature over time, and personal insights are properly assimilated into respective areas of life, we are unlikely to experience relapse or any form of mental, emotional, physical, or spiritual regression.

When recovery principles and yogic practices are brought together, we appreciate the miracle of life and fulfill our individual and collective destinies. We are empowered to think, say, and do what we need to think, say, and do in the reality of now. We discover how to evolve at our own pace, let go of things that no longer serve our highest good, and awaken to new levels of consciousness. We comprehend that we are an essential part of the unfoldment of the universe, which means we know when, where, and how to offer love and service in every situation throughout each day.

YOU ARE THE FUTURE OF RECOVERY

Whatever you do to enhance your understanding of recovery and yoga, your endeavors will help you now and in your future, and upcoming generations will also benefit. When you individualize and modernize the principles and practices of recovery and yoga, and apply these things to your design for living, your efforts to help others will be productive as you will speak to those in active addiction or recovery with words they understand.

You will inspire and connect with these people because you will recognize in them the very things you have overcome as they recognize in you the very things they wish to nurture within their lives. They will believe and trust your message of liberation and redemption because you will offer them something experiential and authentic. They will sense from your peaceful yet powerful presence that you have done the necessary work to change your life, that you are actively continuing to accomplish great things, and that you are capable of passing along that which will equip them to make things right in their lives. They will see that you are a living example of healing and hope, strength and grace, empathy and transformation. They will want what you have and they will do what you suggest—so long as your commitment to your program of action remains strong and your approach to sharing your truth remains heart centered and service oriented.

You are destined to be a hero in recovery. After you learn how to save and improve your own life, you will get to help others do the same. When you step onto this path of revitalization, forge ahead with conviction, humility, and gratitude. Advance always toward a brighter future for yourself and all human beings. Continue to explore your spiritual practices, learn to offer greater sympathy to all living things, do the best you can with what you know within the reality of now, and trust that your conception of God or a higher power of your own understanding will direct, guide, and protect you as you bring light where there is darkness, kind words where there are uncomfortable silences, and smiles and warm embraces wherever there is loneliness or despair.

A MANTRA FOR SUCCESS

Below is a yogic mantra to invoke peace, wisdom, and prosperity in your life. It removes obstacles, negativity, and fear so that success is ensured. It is renowned for its ability to awaken one's inner virtues and release blocked energies within the mind and body—enabling one to feel grounded and secure and benefit all humankind with one's thoughts, speech, and actions.

Om gam ganapataye namaha

Chant this mantra silently or aloud. Repeat it as many times as you like. Sing along with a recorded rendition. Use a mala bead necklace if you have one, and touch each bead as you chant. Be devotional or intentional. Believe the mantra will calm your mind and harmonize your body. Believe it will clear a pathway for you. Believe it will anchor your awareness in the here and now. Believe it will give you knowledge and power so that you can be the person you are here to be.

LET'S CONTINUE OUR JOURNEY TOGETHER

To further explore the concepts in this book, consider listening to my audio courses "Recovery: Principles for a Purposeful Life," "Yogic Principles for Transformation," and "Yogic Wisdom for Modern Times" on Insight Timer. These courses feature supplemental teachings, personal stories, and an interactive community classroom where I reply to all questions and comments and offer personalized suggestions to support you on your journey.

From my heart to yours, thank you for being
here.
May you know love and happiness, freedom
and peace.
I am with you in spirit always.
Namaste.

ACKNOWLEDGMENTS

Anna Dioguardi for being my first yoga teacher nearly two decades ago in NYC. Thank you for singing such sweet songs during *savasana*.

Chelsey Charbeneau for being my first yoga teacher in Los Angeles and for being my friend. Thank you for telling me I would be a yoga teacher someday and that I would write a book about my experiences.

Arune K., you were the first person I talked to when I knew I needed to stop drinking. You listened with compassion. I will never forget your support and friendship.

John F. for picking me up and taking me to twelve-step meetings in West Hollywood. You helped me get my first "Big Book" at the Log Cabin. You taught me not to "compare and despair" and that recovery happens "when one alcoholic talks with another."

Joe F. for continuing to ask me if I wanted to work the twelve steps until I finally said yes. You saved my life.

Troy A., Durk J., Joe R., and all the men at the P&G group. I learned how to think, speak, and act by listening at those meetings. You also taught me how to make and keep commitments.

Nate B. for allowing me to walk you through all twelve steps. This is one of my favorite memories from my early recovery.

Navah for our therapy sessions during my first six months of sobriety. You created a safe space for me to try to articulate my thoughts and feelings so I could find my authentic voice.

Jan B. for asking me to help you get sober and for letting me do my best to share my experience, strength, and hope with you.

Leon B. for sending inspirational text messages to me (and countless others) every morning. Those spiritual quotes helped me start each day with a smile.

Maury S. for reaching out when I was a newcomer. We have developed our friendship for more than a dozen years now. It is a privilege to walk this path with you. I consider you my brother.

Tommy R. for being a living example of yoga and recovery. I remember visiting your house in Venice while you were writing your book. You gave me my first opportunities to teach yoga to people in recovery. Thank you for lighting a path so I could see where I was headed.

Kevin J. for taking my phone calls and helping me through a geographical transition when I was three years sober.

Hans L., Brooke B., Colin S., and Peter G. for inviting me into the Artist's Way group. Thank you for sharing your truths and talents and for letting me share mine.

Mike A. for being an angel in my life. We have walked this road together for nearly a decade now. Thank you for helping me through a major life transition when I was seven years sober. And thank you for living your program with such humility and selflessness.

Dan M., I found you at the perfect time to help me work on a part of my life that needed transformation. You helped me do that and I am forever grateful.

Saul David Raye, thank you for showing me how to teach yoga from my heart. Namaste.

Maty Ezraty, thank you for exemplifying how to honor the seat of the teacher. May your spirit rest in peace always.

Molly D. for helping me establish a relationship with Cliffside Malibu where I have taught thousands of yoga classes.

The team at Insight Timer: Maddy Gerrard for inviting me to share my guided meditations. Tash Slavec for suggesting I create a course about addiction recovery. Isabelle Pikorn for publishing my articles about yogic philosophy.

My sister Michele, you are always there for me. You are a great teacher and fantastic mother. I love you.

My brother Rick, I wish you the best now and forever. Your kids are lucky to have you as a dad. I love you.

My father, Irv, thank you for the gift of life. I hope you are proud of what I have done with it so far. I love you.

My mother, Jann, your spirit guides me from heaven. This book would not have been possible without your presence in my heart. I love you.

Shambhala Publications, especially my editor, Beth Frankl. Thank you for your interest in helping me share my professional and personal experience with recovery and yoga. Thank you for your suggestion to add more yogic philosophy; the creative freedom I was given; the deadline extensions; and for turning my manuscript into a book that may be helpful to those in need for years to come. Special thanks to Peter Schumacher for guiding the manuscript through various editorial stages, and to Ashley Benning for such thoughtful and thorough copyediting.

My literary agent, Rita Rosenkranz. Thank you for believing in me and my work from the very beginning. Thank you for helping me format my proposal and sending it out on my behalf, reading our contract and advocating for my best interests, and your unwavering reliability and professionalism.

Sandra, thank you for the most precious gift, our daughter.

My Lilia Jewel, I love you more than I can express in words. You are here in this world to do amazing things. You give my life real purpose, and it is an honor to be your father. I am here for you now and forevermore. You are my best teacher.

RESOURCES FOR RECOVERY

Al-Anon: al-anon.org

Alcoholics Anonymous: aa.org

Anorexics and Bulimics Anonymous: aba12steps.org

Cocaine Anonymous: ca.org

Debtors Anonymous: debtorsanonymous.org

Depression and Bipolar Support Alliance: dbsalliance.org

Gamblers Anonymous: gamblersanonymous.org

Narcotics Anonymous: na.org

National Association for Children of Addiction: nacoa.org

National Institute on Drug Abuse: nida.nih.gov

Overdose Lifeline: overdoselifeline.org

Overeaters Anonymous: oa.org

Partnership to End Addiction: drugfree.org

SAMHSA (Substance Abuse and Mental Health Services
    Administration) National Helpline: 1-800-662-HELP (4357);
    samhsa.gov
Sex and Love Addicts Anonymous: slaafws.org
Suicide and Crisis Lifeline: 988lifeline.org
Veterans Crisis Line: veteranscrisisline.net

SUGGESTED READING

Alcoholics Anonymous World Services, Inc. *Daily Reflections.*
New York: Alcoholics Anonymous World Services, Inc., 2014.

Allen, James. *The Complete James Allen Collection.* San
Bernardino, CA: The Best Books Publishing, 2019.

Barks, Coleman. *The Essential Rumi.* San Francisco: Harper,
1995.

Easwaran, Eknath, trans. *The Bhagavad Gita.* Berkeley, CA: The
Blue Mountain Center of Meditation, 2007.

———. *The Dhammapada.* Berkeley, CA: The Blue Mountain
Center of Meditation, 2007.

———. *The Upanishads.* Berkeley, CA: The Blue Mountain
Center of Meditation, 1987.

Dalai Lama, His Holiness the Fourteenth. *Beyond Religion*. London: Random House, 2012.

———. *The Good Heart*. New York: Simon and Schuster, 2016.

Fox, Emmet. *Alter Your Life*. San Francisco: Harper San Francisco, 1994.

———. *Around the Year with Emmet Fox: A Book of Daily Readings*. San Francisco: Harper San Francisco, 1992.

———. *Make Your Life Worthwhile*. New York: HarperCollins, 1946.

———. *Power through Constructive Thinking*. San Francisco: Harper & Row, 1990.

———. *The Sermon on the Mount*. London: HarperCollins, 2010.

Gandhi, Mahatma. *The Way to God*. Berkeley, CA: Berkeley Books, 1999.

Griffiths, Bede. *The Marriage of East and West*. Springfield, IL: Templegate, 1982.

———. *Return to the Center*. Springfield, IL: Templegate, 1976.

Hazelden. *Came to Believe: The Spiritual Adventure of A.A. As Experienced by Individual Members*. New York: Alcoholics Anonymous World Services, Inc., 1973.

Ladinsky, Daniel. *The Gift: Poems by Hafiz, the Great Sufi Master*. London: Penguin, 1999.

Lawrence, Brother. *The Practice of the Presence of God*. Grand Rapids, MI: Revell, 1967.

Merton, Thomas. *Contemplative Prayer*. London: Darton, Longman & Todd, 2005.

———. *Life and Holiness*. New York: Herder and Herder, 1963.

———. *Spiritual Direction & Meditation*. Collegeville, MN: Liturgical Press, 1960.

Nhat Hanh, Thich. *The Art of Communicating*. New York: HarperOne, 2014.

——. *Happiness: Essential Mindfulness Practices*. New York: Penguin Random House, 2005.

——. *The Miracle of Mindfulness: An Introduction to the Practice of Meditation*. London: Beacon Press, 1987.

——. *Peace Is Every Step: The Path of Mindfulness in Everyday Life*. New York: Bantam, 1992.

——. *Reconciliation: Healing the Inner Child*. Berkeley, CA: Parallax Press, 2010.

——. *Teachings on Love*. Berkeley, CA: Parallax Press, 1997.

Oliver, Mary. *Devotions: The Selected Poems of Mary Oliver*. New York: Penguin Press, 2017.

——. *Dream Work*. Boston: Atlantic Monthly Press, 1986.

Prabhavananda, Swami. *Sermon on the Mount According to Vedanta*. New York: Vedanta Society of Southern California, 1992.

Teresa, Mother. *No Greater Love*. Novato, CA: New World Library, 1989.

Tolle, Eckhart. *A New Earth: Awakening to Your Life's Purpose*. New York: Dutton/Penguin Group, 2005.

——. *The Power of Now: A Guide to Spiritual Enlightenment*. Novato, CA: New World Library, 1999.

Vivekananda, Swami. *Jnana-Yoga*. New York: Ramakrishna-Vivekananda Center, 1955.

——. *Raja-Yoga*. New York: Ramakrishna-Vivekananda Center, 1956.

Wilson, Bill. *Alcoholics Anonymous: The Big Book,* 4th ed. New York: Alcoholics Anonymous World Services, Inc., 2002.

———. *The Language of the Heart: Bill W.'s Grapevine Writings.* New York: AA. Grapevine, Inc., 1988.

———. *Twelve Steps and Twelve Traditions.* New York: Alcoholics Anonymous World Services, Inc., 2012.

Yogananda, Paramahansa. *In the Sanctuary of the Soul: A Guide to Effective Prayer.* Los Angeles: Self-Realization Fellowship Press, 1998.

———. *Metaphysical Meditations.* Los Angeles: Self-Realization Fellowship Press, 1994.

———. *The Yoga of Jesus.* Los Angeles: Self-Realization Fellowship Press, 2007.

ABOUT THE AUTHOR

Brian Hyman is an accomplished, certified yoga therapy teacher with more than a dozen years of personal recovery from addiction and over ten years of professional experience facilitating thousands of yoga classes, meditation sessions, and process groups at Cliffside Malibu, a prominent treatment center for addiction recovery in Malibu, California.

Brian has written articles about recovery, yoga, and spirituality for *Whole Life Times*, *Mantra Wellness + Health*, *Yoga Digest*, *Origin*, *role/reboot*, *Upward Frog*, and *Best You Ever*. He has been interviewed about his innovative and dedicated work by *Voyage LA*, *Shoutout LA*, *Neon Tommy*, *Malibu Times Magazine*, *Recovery 2.0*, *The Acorn*, *Heroes in Recovery*, and *Sivana Spirit*. He has shared his insightful and experiential perspective about addiction, healing, and transformation on the podcasts *Sober Gratitudes*, *Sobriety Corps*, *Stories of Inspiring Joy*, and *Yoga And*... His yoga classes, breathing tutorials, and guided meditations were featured for many years on Yoga30, and his course "Meditation for Everyone: Calm, Balance, and Peace" has been completed by thousands of students around the world on Udemy.

Brian has served as a yoga ambassador for lululemon, Manduka, Yoga Aid, and Yoga Earth to help raise awareness and funds for causes that support people in need. He also helped make yoga accessible and affordable for many years in Los Angeles by organizing and teaching free and donation-based weekly classes, including 12-Step Yoga (West Hollywood), Strand Street Yoga (Santa Monica), and Yoga for Recovery (Agoura Hills).

Brian is the creator of the thirty-day audio course "Recovery: Principles for a Purposeful Life" on Insight Timer. His other courses on this platform include "Cultivating a Heart of Gratitude," "Yogic Principles for Transformation," "Yogic Wisdom for Modern Times," "Finding Happiness & Inner Peace," "Understanding the Twelve Steps," "Dharma of Recovery: 5 Powers," "Dharma of a Rope: Seeing Things Clearly," and "Dharma of a Flower: Awakening in the Here and Now." These recordings, in addition to his guided meditations, total more than a million plays altogether worldwide.

For more information, visit brianhymanyoga.com.